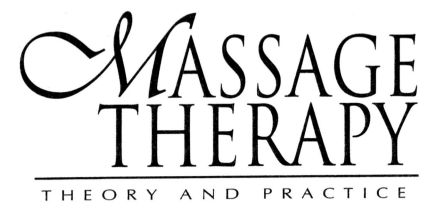

MASSAGE THERAPY

THEORY AND PRACTICE

Jean E. Loving, BA, LMT
Seminar Network International, Inc.
Lake Worth, Florida

Pearson
Education

Appleton & Lange
Stamford, Connecticut

Healing Mechanisms of the Body 22
Pain and Inflammation Processes 25
Physiological Effects of Massage 28
Psychological Effects of Massage 33
Emotional and Spiritual Effects of Massage 34
Current Research 35
Indications for Massage 35
Contraindications for Massage 37
Special Populations 38
Endangerment Sites 38
Referrals 41
Review Questions 42

Chapter 4.   Sanitation, Safety, and Personal Hygiene 43
Learning Objectives 43
Vocabulary Terms 43
Introduction 44
Microorganisms and Common Diseases 44
Sanitation Practices 47
Special Conditions for Massage Therapists 49
Safety Practices and Accident Prevention 50
Personal Hygiene 50
Review Questions 51

Chapter 5.   The Science and Art of Massage 53
Learning Objectives 53
Vocabulary Terms 54
Introduction 54
Body, Mind, Spirit Connection 54
The Mainstream Approach 56
The Energetic Approach or Model 57
Mainstream Medical Approach and Energetic
    Approach 59
Postural Assessment/Body Reading 59
Current Research 60
Case Studies 65
Review Questions 67

**Chapter 6.   Preparation for and Consultation with
    the Client** 69
Learning Objectives 69
Vocabulary Terms 70
Atmosphere for Massage 70
Determining the Client's Needs 72
Client–Therapist Interaction 73
Palpation Skills 76

Developing a Treatment Plan 76
Positioning and Draping the Client 77
After the Massage 79
Review Questions 80

Chapter 7.   Major Massage Strokes 81
Learning Objectives 81
Vocabulary Terms 81
Introduction 82
The Seven Basic Massage Strokes 82
Application of Basic Massage Strokes 93
Proprioception in Body Tissue 110
Stretching and Lengthening 113
Contemporary Therapeutic Massage Approaches 115
Case Studies 123
Review Questions 124

**Chapter 8.   Contemporary Therapeutic Massage
Approaches** 125
Learning Objectives 125
Vocabulary Terms 126
Introduction 126
Cranial–Sacral Therapy 126
Connective Tissue Therapies or Fascial
    Techniques 127
Fascial Kinetics (Bowen Technique) 129
Manual Lymphatic Drainage Massage or
    Vodder Lymph Drainage 129
Muscle Energy Techniques .131
Myofascial Techniques 137
Neuromuscular Techniques 139
Oriental Therapies 149
Seated Massage 159
Structural Alignment and Postural Integration
    Techniques 160
Vibrational Therapies or Energy Therapy 161
Learning and Integrating Approaches 170
Case Studies 171
Review Questions 171

**Chapter 9.   Assessment: Designing the Massage to Fit
the Client** 173
Learning Objectives 173
Vocabulary Terms 174
Introduction 174
Assessment 174

Special Tests 176
Routines 178
Quick Assessment Tools for Case Studies 178
Case Studies 180
Review Questions 184

**Chapter 10.   Self-Care and Wellness for Therapist
and Client** 185
Learning Objectives 185
Vocabulary Terms 186
Stress and Tension 186
Student and Massage Therapist Burnout 187
Activities and Exercises for Self-Care 189
Review Questions 209

**Chapter 11.   Therapeutic Massage: The Application
of Knowledge to Client Needs** 211
Learning Objectives 211
Vocabulary Terms 212
General Pathologies and Massage Treatments 212
Use of Hydrotherapy and Spa Treatments 216
Components for Adapting Massage
to Specific Treatments 225
Specific Treatments 225
Special Populations 240
Case Studies 244
Review Questions 247

Appendix A.   Case Studies 249

Appendix B.   Code of Ethics 251

Appendix C.   Client Folder Forms 255

Appendix D.   Pregnancy Routine and Infant Massage 261

Appendix E.   SOAP Notes With Six Massage Routines 265

Appendix F.   Resource and Information List 273

Bibliography 277

Glossary 281

Index 291

FOREWORD

I have had the pleasure of knowing and working with Jean Loving since the late 1980s when we sat on a committee together pondering the future of massage therapy. Massage has come a long way since then, thanks in part to people like Jean, who are making an effort to pass on the breadth and depth of their knowledge to others in the field.

Jean is the daughter of teachers and was immersed in a rich learning environment as a child. From this, she developed her joy of reading, her lifelong pursuit of personal growth and character building, and her interest in connecting cultures and people. She has traveled to and lived in various parts of the world with her husband and four children. Her cultural experiences and interests are evident in her writing.

Following in her parents' footsteps, Jean became a teacher and taught for many years in Canada and the United States. She especially loves teaching adult learners and helping them develop self-directed learning skills that enable them to take responsibility for their lives.

Jean is unique among massage therapists because of her background in both education and massage. She brings to her teaching sound educational principles, a wealth of life experience, and many years of massage practice. Out of this exceptional combination comes her book, *Massage Therapy: Theory and Practice.*

With this book, Jean makes a critical contribution to the body of massage knowledge. By providing learning objectives and vocabulary terms at the beginning of each chapter, she enables the reader to integrate and synthesize the material even as it is being read. At the end of each chapter she redirects the reader's attention to the material by providing review questions. This is especially helpful for adult learners, who have conflicting priorities while in school. Jean also provides the opportunity for continued study by thoroughly documenting the information in her book.

Jean takes a comprehensive approach to educating the reader. She leads the way through an assortment of worthwhile themes like the history of massage, effects and benefits, indications and contraindications, client management, basic and demanding techniques, ethics, and meeting client needs. The inclusion of topics like hygiene and self-care ensures that massage therapists will understand how to stay healthy while maintaining a busy practice.

Although new students will find it an excellent resource, *Massage Therapy: Theory and Practice* is not just for beginners. Jean challenges massage therapists who have been in the field to refine their knowledge and embrace massage as both a science and an art. This book affords the reader an opportunity to see massage therapy through the eyes of someone who has a unique perspective on the field. For those interested in greater wisdom and expanded insight, Jean's book is a gift.

Sally Niemand
Northern Lights School of Massage Therapy

ACKNOWLEDGMENTS

I wish to thank the many people in my life who have encouraged me—sometimes by their example and sometimes by the subject matter being taught. I am grateful, too, for the family members, colleagues, and friends who often took over duties to allow me to complete this book. I especially wish to thank Larry Loving, my husband of 47 years, who as usual spent many hours on the computer, editing and helping me to finish this project.

In the production of this book, I thank all those who contributed to the manuscript, particularly my editor, Kimberly Davies, for her interest, support, and editorial help. Thank yous are also extended to Lisa M. Guidone, Production Editor, Eve Siegel, Art Coordinator, and Wendy Jackelow for her illustrations.

Finally, I thank all those who have been my students or students with me through the years. Many hours of my life have been spent teaching and learning, and each student along the way has added something to my life. They have been my greatest teachers.

I am eternally grateful to all.

Jean E. Loving
1998

INTRODUCTION

Twelve years ago, when I left public education, I knew little about where the massage world would take me. After graduating from a leading massage school, I developed a practice doing structural alignment work with injured clients. After that, I worked with a variety of osteopaths and chiropractors, began teaching at a local massage school, and eventually took it over. The school became successful and I branched out in my teaching, instructing others across the United States and Canada in an eclectic form of structural alignment. During my years of teaching at the massage school, I recognized the need for a textbook that went beyond the basic massage books available. The massage student needs help integrating modalities and putting current theory and knowledge into practice. This book is dedicated to that end. I am extremely grateful to this profession and I hope that, in some small way, the writing of this book will help others along similar paths.

This book is aimed at those students and schools where time or inclination allows the student not only to master but to go beyond Swedish massage. Several very good books are available to assist the student in mastering Swedish massage. It is my hope that dedicated educators will apply the other techniques treated in this book so that the many modalities now practiced in the United States and Canada can be integrated with basic Swedish massage.

Practitioners performing massage should consider a holistic approach that integrates all aspects of body, mind, emotions, and spirit. The extent of therapeutic benefits our clients receive depends largely upon this approach. Traditionally, the medical community has not embraced this holistic approach, and as a result, it is necessary to bring some of the medical approach to the creative, artistic side of massage. So you will find both elements in this book. This idea is to balance both approaches. After all, human beings have been endowed with both a left and a right hemisphere of the brain. Not only do we want to see logical, process-oriented, time-limited massage when called for, we also want to see a creative, intuitive, "I know this is right" massage without always understanding why and how. An integration of Eastern and Western thought will allow massage therapy to address the energy systems of the body as well as the physiological body.

I believe that a core body of knowledge must be recognized by school owners and students so that the profession may grow and prosper. A certain level of standardization will be required. In massage vocabulary, for instance, it is standard practice to use the term "therapist," but it is unclear which term, "patient" or "client," is more appropriate. For the purposes of this book, "client" will be used. Those not comfortable with this word may substitute "patient" as they read along.

Another issue that needs clarification is the number of hours needed by a student to complete a basic training program. With the onset of the National Certification Exam pegged at 500 hours, the issue is clearer; however, many programs do not meet this criterion.

In Canada, the standard training required to become a Registered Massage Therapist ranges from 2600 to 3000 hours. To my knowledge, no school in the United States offers this level of basic training. Moreover, many schools have had to add courses and modalities to encourage additional training after basic training is finished. Educators need to improve the training of massage therapists. Many massage therapy schools are doing this, but we have a long way to go before we match our Canadian cousins or other medically trained personnel in the various allied health fields similar to massage in the United States. I hope this book becomes a stepping stone in achieving this goal.

1

PHILOSOPHY AND HISTORY OF MASSAGE

In 800 BC, Homer reported in the Odyssey *that war-worn heroes were massaged with perfumed oil to rest and refresh.*

LEARNING OBJECTIVES

After reading this chapter, students will be able to:
1. Discuss the development of massage from its roots to the present day.
2. Discuss the meaning of the root words of "massage."
3. Describe the origins of Swedish massage.
4. Follow the development of current trends in massage through history.
5. Project trends in massage based on current thought.
6. Discuss several massage therapies in use in the United States today.
7. Define the following vocabulary terms.

VOCABULARY TERMS

Massage	Swedish massage	Tsubos
Shaman		

▪ INTRODUCTION

The past, present, and future are connected, much like the links of a chain. The chain provides the structure or whole; each link is separate and unique.

By studying the development of massage through time, we have a sense of the whole profession—where it came from, where it is today, and hints of where it is going tomorrow. Someone once asked the great philosopher Santayana why history should be studied, and his reply was "to learn from the past." If we do not learn from the past, we repeat it.

Today, massage therapy stands on its own as a profession within the healthcare community. It is closely aligned with the medical field, performed in hospitals on patients and staff in several U.S. cities and states as well as in European and Chinese facilities; in doctors' and chiropractors' offices; in birthing centers and rehabilitation clinics; and sometimes in private practices and as part of the outreach programs of massage schools. Yet massage is also performed in health spas and massage clinics, on the athletic field, and in homes and offices. These latter incidences show massage as an ally to the healthcare field. Whenever and however it is performed—by physicians, professional massage therapists, practitioners, or students—it is a valued enhancement to health.

Just as massage today is done all over the globe, it has origins in several cultures. The definition of **massage** today is somewhat broader than its root meanings. (See Box 1–1.) The modern term began to appear in European and American writings around 1875. It was referred to as using the hands to manipulate the soft tissues of the body, and generally meant **Swedish massage,** a Western style of massage. It used the French terms for the five strokes: *effleurage*, *pettrisage*, *friction*, *vibration*, and *tapotement*. Today, touch is often added, including the assessment of tissues, manipulation of soft tissue, use of hydrotherapy techniques as adjunct treatments, and helping the client to improve his or her "wellness" state. Massage also includes joint movements and stretching.

▪ HISTORY OF MASSAGE

Long before recorded history, cave dwellers probably rubbed injuries, soothed hurts, and comforted each other when ill. Reaching out to another person through

BOX 1–1   ORIGINS OF THE WORD "MASSAGE"

Latin root *massa* means to squeeze or knead.
Greek root *masso, massein* means to touch, handle, squeeze, or knead.
French verb *masser* means to knead.
Arabic root *mass, mass'h* means to press softly.
Sanskrit word *makeh* means to press softly.

touch is one of the oldest and most fundamental ways humans communicate with each other and care for those injured or ill.

As time went on, hunters and gatherers brewed teas and rubbed herbs and other natural products on the body to alleviate aches and pains. Even in many indigenous cultures today, the herbalist or **shaman** (a healer who combined both doctor and priest roles) is an essential member of the community because of his or her knowledge and ability to promote health.

The natives of Polynesian islands have used massage under various names: on the Sandwich Islands, "lomi lomi"; by the Maoris of New Zealand, "romi romi"; and on Tonga, "toogi toogi." All of these have been practiced since ancient times.

References to massage in literature go back to ancient times. In China, some 4000 years ago, *The Yellow Emperor's Internal Canon* describes massage for healing. As trade between China and the rest of Asia and Europe along the Silk Road increased, ideas were probably taken from one culture to another and became popular. In Japan, rubbing first became amna and more recently shiatsu. In Thailand, joint movement and exercise (Nuad-Bo-Ran) was and still is done in connection with Buddhist temples. In India, rubbing was also used in connection with religious ceremonies; cleaning rituals developed into a form of medicine known as Ayurvedic medicine with origins thousands of years BC. In Persian and Egyptian cultures, aromatic baths and oils were used along with massage and exercises.

In classical Greek culture, massage flourished. The physician, Aesculapius, was known as the god of healing in Greek mythology because of his use of massage in healing. Hippocrates (460–377 BC), known as the father of medicine, described the benefits of using oils and massage on joints as well as exercise. Physicians through the ages have affirmed the phrase "do no harm," which is attributed to Hippocrates. Two other physicians, Diocles of Athens and Galenus (or Galen, 130–200 AD), physician to the gladiators, wrote on the use of manual medicine, exercise, and therapeutic bathing as preventive treatments. In the Greek countryside, the ruins of healing centers such as Epidourous can be seen today. A large, white, circular building containing rooms for health activities, stone massage tables, and resting niches in the walls proved a popular place for citizens. The wide roads, lined with olive trees, that lead into the amphitheatre and "spa" building conjure up ancient pilgrims on foot, in donkey carts, and on crutches, jamming the roadside leading to this healing center. Large bas-relief friezes along the tops of other magnificent ancient buildings depict daily life in ancient Greece. There, among other daily scenes, are people massaging each other, even a youth massaging an adult's leg. Certain Greek and Roman scholars believe the athletes were also receiving massage during their training.

Massage was also part of daily life in the ancient Roman empire. In Pompeii, the ruins include large Roman bath houses with pools for varied baths and large stone massage tables, worn deep with body shapes, sitting in the middle of rooms. A wealthy man had his slave attend to him at the bath, oiling the body and scraping off the oil and dirt accumulated in past days. Next came a massage and finally the various available baths. A poor man oiled and scraped himself down. Among the professionals offering services at the baths were doctors, barbers, hair pluckers, trainers, and masseurs (Balsdon, 1969). Baths were common elsewhere. Seneca

(4 BC–65 AD) reported that living above the baths was very noisy. He could hear the smacks as the masseurs hit their patients. One sound was flat as the hand hit flat on the shoulders. Another sound was hollow, as in cupping (Paoli, 1967).

Bas-reliefs on large buildings elsewhere in Rome depict people giving massage to each other. Julius Caesar himself was reported to have a pinching technique treatment regularly to relieve his neuralgia and epilepsy. The historian Pliny (61–113 AD) was rubbed for relief of asthma. Dr. Aulus Celsus (25 BC–50 AD) wrote an encyclopedia of medicine and talked about massage as preventive treatment for headaches, fever, and paralysis. Numerous gladiatorial schools in Rome and elsewhere prepared men for the games of combat used for private as well as public entertainment. Doctors, trainers, and masseurs were part of the staff involved in the training (Balsdon, 1969). As the Roman culture spread throughout the known world, massage practices were absorbed into many cultures. The Roman culture spread as far north as northern England where, at Bath, a Roman spa is a current tourist attraction.

In Turkey and the former Yugoslavia, the remains of once-great civilizations can still be seen. Remnants of spas like Pamukkale in Turkey, where sparkling mineral water flows around and over giant columns from an earlier time, still entice tourists to spend their holidays there. King Darius of Persia (d. 404 BC) is reported to have spent winters at this site, as did Hadrian and his army. In his book, *Canon of Medicine*, the Persian physician Avicenna (980–1037) recommended massage for babies and the elderly. A Moor from Spain, Averros (1126–1198) integrated Islamic and Greek thought in writing about medicine and massage. The Persian philosopher Rhazes (or Razi) (860–932 AD) was a follower of Hippocrates and Galen and wrote several books on the use of exercise, diet, and massage in the prevention and treatment of disease.

During the Middle Ages (1200–1700 AD), little was written about massage. In Europe, feudal knights and kings endured long winters without battles; the warmer climates to the south in France, Italy, and Spain drew them to spas and cleansing rituals known as "the cure." Bathing, drinking natural mineral waters, and receiving massage most likely prepared them for another year of war and hard living. One such spa still in existence today is in Baden-Baden, Germany. Mary, Queen of Scots, was treated in the 1500s for typhus with massage and she recovered. Often, those suffering from arthritis and rheumatism made yearly trips to southern European spas. Spa treatment consisted of mineral baths, drinking mineral waters, exercise, and massage. A few names have survived from this era. In the 1500s and 1600s, Paracelsus in Switzerland; Ambroise Paré, a surgeon in France; and Prospero Alpinus in Italy used friction strokes and rubbing techniques in treatments. By the middle of the 1700s, massage reached most European countries. In some cultures like the Scandinavian countries and Slavic nations, it survived the earlier hardship of being seen as superstitious and became associated with the mainstream medical community.

Today, in many European and Oriental cultures, massage is received in hospitals, performed by specially trained individuals or physicians and prescribed by doctors as part of their regular medical treatments. Examples include the lymphatic drainage technique and the hydrotherapies done in Austria and Germany. In China, the various components of massage (Chi Gong exercises, herbals, acupuncture, and massage) merged into what is now known as Traditional Chinese Medicine (TCM).

Today, Chinese physicians first train in Western methods and then in TCM. A massage trip to China taken by 32 U.S. therapists confirmed these practices in 9 hospitals visited in 1989. The author was among this group. In China, massage is performed in hospitals and done by physicians. Figure 1–1 shows the use of massage in a Chinese hospital setting today.

The development of the modern system of Swedish massage is attributed to Per Henrik Ling (1776–1839), a professor and physiologist in Stockholm. He had access to earlier letters written from China by Jesuits and began to create, develop, and practice a system of massage movements. He taught these movements at the Stockholm University to gymnasts and physicians, and he was given a special award for his work by the King of Sweden.

In 1813, Ling established the Royal Swedish Central Institute of Gymnastics, where his movements were known as active exercise, resistive exercise duplicated (by the client), and passive stretching. Today, we would call them range-of-motion movements or stretching massage. His system spread throughout Europe, primarily through the many physicians he taught and his successors. The Ling system (called Swedish movements or the movement cure) was often taught in classes lasting 6 to 7 hours per day and over a 3-year period. Within several years of his death, institutes that taught his methods were established in Denmark and Russia. Mathias Roth, an English physician who studied under Ling, published the first book in English on the system and established the first institution in England to teach the methods. Charles Fayette Taylor, one of the Taylor brother physicians, became a student

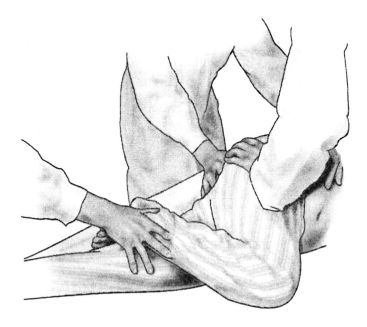

FIGURE 1–1. Patient receiving treatment in a Chinese hospital setting.

of Roth and introduced the methods to the United States. The other Taylor brother, George Henry, went to Stockholm and learned the techniques there. Both men wrote and published articles and textbooks in the United States that advanced massage in both the public and medical fields.

The Art of Massage, by John H. Kellogg (1895), medical director of Battle Creek Sanitarium, noted seven strokes of massage including touch and joint movements. His uses for massage included displacement of many visceral organs and treatments for sciatic nerve syndrome, rheumatism, and fractures.

From the late 1700s to early 1800s, massage developed in many European countries. In Holland, Dr. J. G. Mezger (1838–1909), a practitioner of massage and teacher, believed massage was essential in the remedial treatment of disease. He treated the Kings of Denmark and Sweden, the Czarina of Russia, and the Empress of Austria, thus furthering the spread of massage in those countries. He preferred the French terms of *effleurage, petrissage,* and *tapotement.* This furthered their use within Swedish massage. The term *massage* was not used in the United States until 1874, when Douglas Graham from Boston wrote about massage and its history and applications. He continued to write and promote massage into the 1900s. In Scotland, William Balfour wrote about the uses of compression and friction (1819). In France, Just Marie Lucas-Champronniere used several massage terms, and in Sweden Enril Andrea Gabriel Kleer (1847–1923) used all of the terms now connected to Swedish massage. In 1900, Albert Hoffa published a book, *Technik der Massage,* in Germany. It gives a clear description of strokes and the basis of modern technique.

A combination of these events meant physicians were studying massage and passing on their knowledge to other physicians. The public and the scientists began to read articles that appeared in magazines and medical journals. As heads of state and well-known individuals received massage, further acceptance by the medical field and the public continued to spread. By the early 1900s, massage, therapeutic baths, and exercise were recommended by physicians in several European countries and appeared in the training of physicians in Germany, Denmark, Sweden, and Norway. It was believed that massage helped ailments such as rheumatism, detoxifying and helping body systems to function more successfully. Institutes to train massage practitioners began to appear in Europe.

Because massage developed either within or connected to the medical field or in the lineage of folk medicine, an uneven quality of education existed in the United States and England by the late 1800s. In 1886, in the United States, Charles Mills criticized both the education and the unsubstantiated claims made by practitioners of massage. Massage scandals erupted in England in 1894 over inconsistent education and practices, improper recruiting practices, and false advertisements. In the same year, however, the first organization was formed by eight masseuses who sought to impose standards on training and the practice of massage. By 1939, their membership reached 12,000, and rigorous exams were given and restrictions put on types of practices. This balancing attempt was only partially successful (Van Why, 1991).

Massage suffered as a result of these scandals and of the added scientific and technological advances of the early 1900s. Electricity brought the invention of vibrators and other electrical devices that took the place of manual treatment. Physicians no longer studied massage. Rather, they endorsed new treatments based on pharmacology and surgeries. Drugs, pills, and surgery took the place of treating disease by diet, massage, and hydrotherapy. Although a decline of massage was evident in the United States in the early 1900s, several trends began to influence massage.

▪ CURRENT THOUGHTS AND TRENDS

Sigmund Freud (1856–1939) and his assistant, Wilhelm Reich, developed psychoanalysis and used massage and hydrotherapy techniques in the treatment of hysteria and the mentally ill. The benefits of reduced stress and relaxed states following massage became known by Reich. He left Austria and came to the United States, where he became interested in what bodywork could do for the patient. Somaticrelease techniques were begun by Reich. Later, Bio-energetics, founded by Alexander Lowen, a student of Reich, expanded his work to include the release of pent-up emotions as well as the release of armoring in the body. As the work of these men became known, the massage field expanded.

During the polio epidemics in the United States and Canada from 1917 to 1918 and again in the early 1950s, Sister Kenny demonstrated how massage was successful in the prevention of paralysis and crippling due to the disease as well as in rehabilitation. After World War I, massage was in great demand, and the Reconstruction Department of the United States Army arranged short, intensive courses to train women to meet this demand. Mary McMillan, who had been trained in England (1911–1915) and was in charge of massage and therapeutics in hospitals there, came to the United States and was put in charge of massage in Children's Hospital in Portland, Maine. Later she became chief aide at Walter Reed Army Hospital. From 1921 to 1925 she was director of physiotherapy courses at Harvard Medical School. In 1932, she wrote *Massage and Therapeutic Exercise,* which became influential in the field of massage.

Another influential woman in Europe in the late 1920s was Elizabeth Dicke. She developed a system of massage known as Bindegewebsmassage in Germany. It is based on the reflex action of the body and referral of related visceral problems, such as headaches, to areas of the back. By treating herself for a circulatory problem in her right leg, she developed this form of connective tissue massage. (Tested by years of clinical study in many parts of Europe, the technique is used both for diagnostic purposes and treatment.) Later, Maria Ebner popularized the system in England, now known as connective tissue massage.

In the mid-1900s, despite these trends, massage was still struggling for recognition. Physical therapy now required licensing, and the forerunner to the American Massage Therapy Association, the American Association of Masseurs and Masseuses, was founded in Chicago in 1943.

Zone therapy, or reflexology, the study and treatment of the feet, was rediscovered by William Fitzgerald in 1913 from ancient Chinese foot massage. Later, Eunice D. Ingham, an advocate of his therapy, continued to teach the method and wrote *Stories the Feet Tell* in 1959.

In Austria, after World War II, Emil Vodder developed manual lymphatic drainage, a system of gentle, rhythmic massage aimed at increasing the functioning of the lymphatic system. Originally taught at the Vodder School in Walches, Austria, manual lymphatic draining is now available in the United States and Canada, and is continuing to grow and develop.

Dr. James Cyriax, an English orthopedic physician, developed deep transverse friction massage. Used on muscles, tendons, and ligaments to treat soft tissue dysfunction, this technique is today one of the main components of connective tissue massage. In 1944, Cyriax wrote *Textbook of Orthopedic Medicine,* now a classic in the study of the dysfunction of soft tissue and joints.

Another resurgence of massage began in the United States around 1960. The medical field's declining use of massage led to its rising use as an alternative approach to wellness. The physical fitness movement, ideas about reducing stress and the prevention of disease, as well as the use of massage on athletes brought massage into the public's awareness again. Bonnie Prudden, author of several books on fitness and control of pain, was a leader in this field. Massage was also aided by the rise of chiropractic care and a renewed interest in acupuncture. Today, many chiropractors use massage techniques in their practices and often employ massage therapists as well.

Two women in the United States have had tremendous influence on massage through their books. *Beard's Massage,* by Gertrude Beard (1964), and *Healing Massage Techniques,* by Frances Tappan (1998, 4th edition), remain standards in the teaching of massage. Both women have devoted years of their lives to the furtherance of massage.

In the 1970s and 1980s, numerous private schools emerged across the nation to teach massage. States began to demand licensure for the practicing of massage. Many associations formed in order for members to share ideas about the development of standards and legislation.

The American Massage Therapy Association (AMTA) advocates the development of standards. The AMTA is the current name of the association founded by graduates of the Chicago Swedish Massage School in 1943. Out of this group, educators and school directors formed, in 1982, the Council of Schools for the purpose of developing and maintaining educational standards across the United States in massage schools. This group took the beginning steps to form an accrediting agency by establishing the Commission on Massage Therapy Approval/Accreditation (COMTAA). In the next few years, standards, policies, and procedures were created and implemented to meet the requirements of the United States Department of Education (USDE). With new developments in the Higher Education Act in 1994, involving philosophy and methods, changes were required to conform to federal requirements. COMTAA is still evolving and more changes may be considered as the group moves toward recognition by the USDE.

Founded in 1992, the National Certification Board for Therapeutic Massage and Bodywork (NCBTMB) is the autonomous governing body for the national certification program and oversees the development and administration of the national certification examination. Its mission is to promote ethics and professionalism by creating and maintaining standards of competency in the field. Certification means that a therapist has met a minimum standard of education and experience in the field of massage therapy and bodywork, displays mastery in five core knowledge areas common to the field, adheres to the NCBTMB's code of ethics, and maintains competency by meeting practice and continuing education requirements for recertification. By December 1996, 22,436 therapists had been certified. In 1992, the first standardized exams were given across the country by the NCBTMB. The exams consist of multiple-choice questions based on the theory and practice of massage, anatomy, physiology, ethics, business practices, and many disciplines of massage such as Rolfing® and Trager®.

At the current time, 24 states license massage practitioners and the length of education has greatly increased. More states are working on licensing therapists and schools, and many state associations are talking about longer courses. In Canada, both Ontario and British Columbia offer 2- and 3-year programs similar to an Allied Health Associate Degree. In the United States, a few programs have moved into community colleges, and one or two university programs are now accepting massage school credits toward a regular degree. In England, the University of Westminster offers degrees in bodywork.

Not everyone, however, wants a professional approach that means more standards, licensing in the states, and more federal government bureaucracy and credentials. The dichotomy of ideas can be read in current massage journals and heard at state association meetings.

If communication remains open among all therapists, our legacies and current thought may come together into a synthesis of the best from everyone and for everyone.

▪ THE FUTURE

Several current thoughts and trends in the field of massage are likely to be amplified in the future. Through history, massage has been aligned at times with the mainstream medical approach of the day. This alignment is likely to become more prevalent as massage moves into hospitals, drug rehabilitation facilities, cancer clinics, and HIV-positive facilities. Some orthopedic and osteopathic physicians known by the author now offer massage through their offices, as do some oncologists. Rehabilitation clinics and pain centers also offer massage. Along with this trend comes the desire for education and for the ability to communicate professionally with physicians and other healthcare practitioners. Also influencing this desire for education is the fact that licensed states and national certification are requiring therapists to continue their learning after their basic course in massage. The number of hours of continuing education required varies from state to state. The National Certification Board now requires 50 hours total over a period of 4 years.

Another trend is the practice of massage in chiropractic offices and clinics. Massage clinics often work closely with lawyers and health insurance companies as well as with other healthcare providers.

Another trend is that massage is often offered in health salons; hair, nail, and tanning salons; private homes; and in places of business. Spas incorporate antistress services and those of fitness as well. Recently, spas have sprung up across the United States and Canada and around the world, often in conjunction with resorts, offering massage therapists another arena for their work. Today, chair massage is being done professionally in airports, malls, corporate offices, large stores, factories, and even on beaches. Clients demonstrate better performance, less stress, fewer injuries, and "feeling better" as a result of weekly massages.

Yet another trend in massage is its use by athletic teams, individual athletes, and at competitions. Often massage is given at charity events, where amateur athletes may experience it for the first time. Some athletic teams travel with their own professional therapists. Other teams contact local therapists in whichever town they perform.

These activities have brought massage to many people. As education continues through television programs, books on massage, home study programs, and magazine articles, more people may take advantage of this healing art.

▪ OVERVIEW OF CURRENT MODALITIES

We will discuss various modalities in later chapters. The following overview will give an idea of the scope and practice of these modalities.

The systems of massage most popular today in the United States and Canada are based on Swedish massage, a bodywork style based on Western massage and hydrotherapy used as a basis for most training programs of massage. Swedish massage consists of five strokes: effleurage, petrissage, friction, vibration, and tapotement (for further detail see Chapter 7). Today these names are often replaced with English words such as *touch, gliding, kneading, friction,* and *percussion.* These strokes can be performed to produce either a sedative or a stimulative massage and can be tailored to the client's individual needs.

In Europe, Swedish massage is often used in conjunction with therapeutic baths and other hydrotherapy techniques in hospitals, as in Germany and Austria. In France, England, and Ireland, Swedish massage is often given in conjunction with beauty therapy treatments and facials.

In China, acupressure-like massage is used to balance the "chi" or energy flow along meridian lines in the body. Most often, as mentioned previously, it is done in hospitals by physicians. A few massage clinics outside the hospital setting are run by blind personnel, with special permission from the government.

In Japan, shiatsu or finger pressure massage is used on pressure points called **tsubos,** and many systems of the body can be affected. Several of the popular shiatsu instructors teaching the modality in the United States today have been trained in Japan.

In Russia, massage follows the mainstream medical approach of Swedish massage, with 48 strokes recognized. Massage is often given in hospitals and is accompanied by hydrotherapy techniques. Rehabilitative massage can and often does use electrical and other machines to aid the patient.

Other massage modalities popular in the United States and Canada include the following. Specialized training is needed for these techniques.

1. *Connective tissue approaches, including myofascial release and cranial–sacral techniques.* All connective tissue approaches are based on mechanically softening the tissue with strokes used to spread and pull the tissue. Once the tissue is loose and soft, it is stretched. This can be done very subtly or on a deep level, depending on the technique and desired outcome.

2. *Lymphatic drainage.* This technique helps to balance the lymphatic system. It has developed from Swedish massage, using light spiral and other movements to speed up the movement of the lymphatic fluids in the body.

3. *Positional release and strain counterstrain.* These approaches use body positioning to elicit physiological responses and neurological and circulatory changes to resolve musculoskeletal dysfunction.

4. *Neuromuscular therapies.* Developed in England in the 1930s and 1940s, neuromuscular therapies today encompass an eclectic combination of trigger point therapy, Trager® approach, reflexology, and others incorporating pain relief, trigger points, nerve entrapment, biomechanics, and stress reduction. These therapies are taught in workshops throughout the United States. Other similar therapies include strain/counterstrain, orthobionomy, and myotherapy. Neuromuscular therapy intervenes in the cycle developed by trauma and/or injury, soft tissue dysfunction, and lack of movement often accompanied by pain.

5. *Oriental techniques.* Amma, tuina, shiatsu, acupressure, jin shin do, Hoshino, Thai massage, and Tibetan point holding are based on the Oriental concepts of meridian lines, chi energy, and creating balance in the body. Some of these therapies are done with the client fully clothed.

6. *Polarity and other energetic approaches.* These systems have been developed based on energetic patterns in the body and can be done with light touch or near touch, just off the body, and are often done over clothing or bed linens.

7. *Structural alignment and postural integration.* Rolfing®, Hellerwork, Pfrimmer Work, SOMA, Neuromuscular Integration and Structural Alignment (NISA), CORE, and Fascial Kinetics have all developed using this idea as their base. These systems began with the development of Rolfing® in the 1940s. Before that, in Germany, Bindegewebsmassage combined the idea of a balanced and coordinated body as a whole, incorporating connective tissue massage and postural alignment.

8. *Integrated approaches.* These approaches all use a variety of methods. In fact, most massages are of this type. The therapist blends the styles he or she knows and designs the massage for the individual client: sports massage, prenatal and infant massage, on-site or seated massage, equine and small animal massage, geriatric massage, Russian massage, and abuse survivor massage are some of those using an integrated approach.

As all of these systems have evolved through the years, many of them overlap in intent, techniques, and outcomes. This is to be expected. Many educators and others interested in a wider view of massage in the United States, for instance, believe that a core body of knowledge should be recognized and passed on to future massage therapists. As the profession moves forward, identifying this core, deciding if and how it will be taught, and determining standards for the profession are topics for discussion and a prime reason for the therapist to be active in local, state, and national associations.

REVIEW QUESTIONS

1. What is the origin of the word "massage"?
2. Name the five strokes of Swedish massage.
3. Describe the origins of Swedish massage.
4. How did massage spread from one culture to another culture?
5. Name an early writer about massage and what he or she wrote about.
6. Where does the phrase, "do no harm," come from?
7. Describe an early spa and the activities that went on there.
8. Describe the four components of Traditional Chinese Medicine still in use in China today.
9. Who is known as the father of Swedish massage?
10. How did the Taylor brothers further the movement of massage in the United States?
11. Describe the contributions of Mary McMillan and Elizabeth Dicke to the massage field.
12. Why are standards for the profession and licensing such an issue today?
13. Name several current trends in massage.
14. What do you think the important issues in massage will be in the future?
15. Discuss several massage therapies used in the United States today.
16. Define the vocabulary terms at the beginning of this chapter.

2

PROFESSIONALISM, LAW, AND ETHICS

There can be no question of holding forth on ethics. I have seen people behave badly with great morality and I note every day that integrity has no need of rules.

Albert Camus

 LEARNING OBJECTIVES

After reading this chapter, students will be able to:
1. Define therapeutic massage.
2. Define scope of practice.
3. Explain why laws, rules, and regulations are needed for governing the practice of massage.
4. Explain why licenses may be revoked.
5. Explain the differences between licenses, diplomas, and certification.
6. Discuss professional codes of ethics, and understand how the practice of good ethics helps to build a successful practice of massage.
7. Define the following vocabulary terms.

VOCABULARY TERMS

Boundaries	Felony	Safe touch
Certification	Informed consent	Scope of practice
Code of ethics	License	Sexual impropriety
Confidentiality	Practitioner	Therapeutic massage
Diploma	Professional demeanor	
Disclosure	Right of refusal	

▪ DEFINITION OF MASSAGE

The definition of massage has changed in parallel to its history. In ancient times, massage simply meant to knead or press. In the mid–1900s, it meant to manipulate the soft tissues of the body. In the early 1980s, massage was defined as the systematic and scientific manipulation of the soft tissues of the body. Today, even that definition is limiting. **Therapeutic massage** today includes assessment, treatment applied by the hands and arms to the various layers and tissues known as soft tissue, many strokes of massage, joint movements (known as range-of-motion movements), and the external use of various forms of hydrotherapy. All of these components are provided for the client in a safe, nonsexual environment. The type, length, and outcome of the treatment is determined jointly by the client and therapist.

Because of the almost limitless ways that massage can now be given, it is difficult to define precisely. The profession itself has a hard time defining it and, in order to be inclusive rather than exclusive, the term "bodywork" has been added to the term "massage" for purposes of this book. This reflects the many types and styles of massage as practiced today.

▪ SCOPE OF PRACTICE

The **scope of practice** of any healthcare provider simply means the limits or boundaries that the law or national standards place upon the way the provider may work or practice. For example, a physician is the only healthcare provider who may diagnose disease or illness and then prescribe medications. A nurse can carry out the physician's directions but cannot diagnose or prescribe. A physician, chiropractor, or trained technician may take x-rays, but a massage therapist may not. In some states a massage therapist may touch a client in order to treat him or her with massage, while other caregivers may not. The type of education, the certificate or diploma received, and the development of national standards by the profession usually define the type of practice a person in healthcare may have. Most healthcare **practitioners** have licenses and certificates that exceed that of the massage therapist. The more education and the higher certificate a person holds, the more the therapist is allowed to do by that profession or by the law.

▪ LICENSING AND LAWS

A state, county, or municipality issues a **license** as a requirement for practicing a trade or profession. In the United States today, the licensing of massage therapists is most often done by the state. Licensing in states developed to protect the public from unregulated massage practice. Some states license healthcare workers to control prostitution. For whatever reason, 24 states now have some form of licensing or registration for massage therapists. It is clear that this trend will continue. Several other states are in the process of creating licensing. Some individual cities and counties within states have passed laws setting certain educational requirements for registration or licensing.

This makes it very difficult for massage therapists to know what the rules and laws are in any particular part of the country. Before you move, check carefully into the requirements of the state, county, or city to which you wish to relocate. The state may have a board of massage; the county a commissioner's office; and the city, the mayor's office, city attorney, or police department, any of which can provide the information you need. (See Box 2–1 for a checklist of licensing information outlets.) If the state does have licensing, it will usually require that you pass the state's examination. Once licensed by the state, you will not need another massage license from the municipality. Massage establishments may also be licensed. Check your local and state authorities. In addition, city occupational license or business laws, zoning laws, and health laws will affect the setup of a massage practice. Be sure to check on all of them.

BOX 2–1   CHECKLIST FOR LICENSING INFORMATION IN YOUR AREA

1. State governmental agencies—For licensing laws, exams, health certificates, department of revenue.
2. County commissioners' offices (if no state license)—For number of hours of education needed, fictitious name registration, insurance requirements, occupational license.
3. City or municipality offices, mayor's office—For business license, local ordinances, advertising, occupational license.
4. Police department—For mug shots, fingerprinting, criminal record searches.
5. County or city planning or zoning board offices—For local business and zoning laws.
6. Local fire department—For safety permit for building.
7. Association or professional organization offices—For educational requirements.
8. Internal Revenue Service—For employer ID number if hiring employees and for resale number if selling products and state tax may be collected.

The reasons given for states to revoke a license once it has been acquired include the following:

- Illegal acts resulting in a **felony,** a major crime.
- An act of prostitution.
- Endangering the health of a client.
- Being addicted to drugs or alcohol.
- Diagnosing or prescribing drugs.
- Illegal advertisements.

Educational Standards

The number of educational hours required by states varies from 250 to 1250 (in Canada, the requirements are 2600–3000 hours). However, the American Massage Therapy Association's (AMTA) and the National Certification Board of Therapeutic Massage and Bodywork's (NCTB) standard of 500 clock hours seems to be accepted as a national standard. Among the subjects studied, it is generally agreed that anatomy and physiology, pathological conditions, massage theory and practice, business practices, ethics, and various modalities are needed for a successful practice. Certainly, consultation with other healthcare professionals is needed when trauma and injury occur. When rehabilitation or hospital care is indicated, then working on a professional healthcare team with direct supervision of the other professionals provides the best care for the client.

One of the main reasons for having a national exam is to standardize state examinations. This would increase the ease of mobility of massage therapists between states. A national certificate will also aid the public in choosing therapists, as requirements become standard between the many types of bodywork providers.

There is a long way to go before all states have licensing, and even then they will not all be similar. A recent symposium sponsored by National Certification Board for Therapeutic Massage and Bodywork spent several days exploring the ideas of standards and professionalism. At the end of the symposium, the majority of those present wanted to continue discussions on this controversial topic. However, there is no clear path ahead. Individuals, associations, and national groups all need to grapple with the ideas of professionalism so that we do become a self-governing body. If we do not regulate ourselves, some other body of professionals will do it for us or to us.

Diplomas and Certification

A **diploma** is granted by an institution to indicate the successful completion of a body of knowledge or a specific program. **Certification** primarily refers to a document presented by the NCBTMB that indicates the successful passing of the National Certification Proficiency Examination. Applicants for the exam must have completed a combination of training programs and practical experience totaling 500 clock hours, must adhere to the NCBTMB Code of Ethics, and must maintain professional competency by meeting practical and continuing education requirements.

Some modality providers or schools issue certification documents when a participant has successfully completed a lengthy training in that modality.

▪ CODE OF ETHICS AND PROFESSIONAL BEHAVIOR

Several professional organizations in massage have created their own codes of ethics for therapists. A **code of ethics** is a standard of professional and acceptable behavior that forms the basis by which people conduct their business. Sometimes the beliefs or values held by one person differ from those held by another. It is difficult to create a value system acceptable to all. For example, one therapist might not want to work on people with cancer or those with other diseases. Another might feel that all persons in need should be treated. In setting up a code of ethics for the profession, both these people and their beliefs may be accommodated.

Codes of Ethics

Code of ethics statements have been put forth by several national associations of massage and by some state associations. Figure 2–1 gives the code of ethics of the American Massage Therapy Association. Appendix B gives the code of ethics of a nationally accredited school of massage therapy and bodywork. Similarities to note between both codes include the following points:

- Commitment to highest-quality care.
- Performing only those services one is qualified to perform.
- Gaining personal and professional growth through continuing education.
- Not engaging in sexual activities with clients.
- Respecting confidentiality of client information.
- Using honesty and integrity in business.

Other code of ethics statements often contain items on draping, respect for client boundaries, and respect for other healthcare professionals. Perhaps you or your class would like to write your own code of ethics and sign it as your commitment to excellence in this, your new profession.

Common Fears and Biases

All massage therapists must explore their own fears, biases, and prejudices about working on clients and face them squarely. If massage therapists are uncomfortable in dealing with clients, clients will also feel it and the treatment will not be in their best interests. Referring a client to another massage therapist is a reasonable solution, providing communication is honest and fair and there is just cause. Usually, it is the student or new massage therapist who voices these fears.

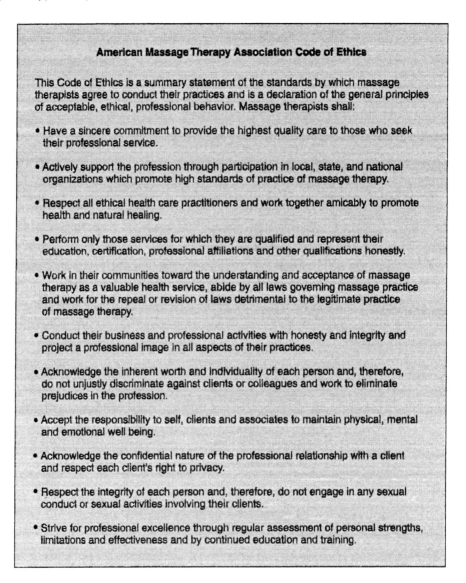

American Massage Therapy Association Code of Ethics

This Code of Ethics is a summary statement of the standards by which massage therapists agree to conduct their practices and is a declaration of the general principles of acceptable, ethical, professional behavior. Massage therapists shall:

• Have a sincere commitment to provide the highest quality care to those who seek their professional service.

• Actively support the profession through participation in local, state, and national organizations which promote high standards of practice of massage therapy.

• Respect all ethical health care practitioners and work together amicably to promote health and natural healing.

• Perform only those services for which they are qualified and represent their education, certification, professional affiliations and other qualifications honestly.

• Work in their communities toward the understanding and acceptance of massage therapy as a valuable health service, abide by all laws governing massage practice and work for the repeal or revision of laws detrimental to the legitimate practice of massage therapy.

• Conduct their business and professional activities with honesty and integrity and project a professional image in all aspects of their practices.

• Acknowledge the inherent worth and individuality of each person and, therefore, do not unjustly discriminate against clients or colleagues and work to eliminate prejudices in the profession.

• Accept the responsibility to self, clients and associates to maintain physical, mental and emotional well being.

• Acknowledge the confidential nature of the professional relationship with a client and respect each client's right to privacy.

• Respect the integrity of each person and, therefore, do not engage in any sexual conduct or sexual activities involving their clients.

• Strive for professional excellence through regular assessment of personal strengths, limitations and effectiveness and by continued education and training.

FIGURE 2–1. Reprinted with permission.

The following is a list of common fears or biases of which the massage therapist should be aware:

• People with communicable diseases. Lack of understanding about transference of the disease is usually the cause.
• Overweight individuals (thought to be undisciplined) or thin people (thought to be obsessive about their appearance).

- Dirty people or people who smell. A simple suggestion is often enough to change this.
- People who have cancer, diabetes, or other diseases. Concern may be legitimate; learn more about the disease and what benefits massage has in that situation, and then seek a physician's approval. This will clarify the situation for you as the therapist.
- People with recent surgeries or ugly scars. Can massage help? If not comfortable, refer to another therapist.
- Same sex or opposite sex massage. Explore and be clear about your reasons. Limit your clientele to those with whom you feel safe.

Some of the terminology used in codes of ethics to describe the relationship between therapist and client is defined as follows:

- **Boundaries.** The client has physical boundaries, invisible barriers that separate the client and therapist, and emotional boundaries that the therapist needs to consider. Receiving permission to enter boundaries is important to the therapist, as mutual trust is the basis of a good client–therapist relationship.
- **Confidentiality.** Client information is private. Sharing client information with anyone without the client's permission will destroy the trust developed between client and therapist.
- **Disclosure.** Reasons for refusing to work with a client must be explained.
- **Informed consent.** The client must have enough information to choose the "right" treatment. The therapist's job is to educate the client.
- **Right of refusal.** The client has the right to stop the treatment or to refuse it at any time.
- **Safe touch.** Touching must be done so that the client experiences no harm or fear. Persons must feel free from harm for trust to be present between therapist and client.
- **Sexual impropriety.** Any behavior, comments, expressions, or gestures that are seductive or sexually demeaning to the client are inappropriate.

Professional Demeanor

Given the stressful times in which we live, the ever-present trend to use lawyers to settle grievances, and the struggle of the profession to achieve higher status in the medical field and with the public, it behooves us to strive for the highest level of professionalism in our business as well as to seek continuous personal growth. We should always present a **professional demeanor,** which refers to the appearance, language, and behavior of practitioners, which meets professional standards and inspires trust and respect.

Some of the qualities that inspire trust and respect might include the following:

Fairness	Human dignity
Integrity and honesty	Patience
Understanding	A service orientation

Knowlege	Quality or excellence
Skill	A capacity for personal growth
Desire	

Perhaps you can add more qualities to this list. The study and application of these powerful qualities and their habits has led many persons to happy, healthy, and successful effectiveness.

REVIEW QUESTIONS

1. Develop a definition for "therapeutic massage" using the components listed in this chapter.
2. Discuss why it is difficult to define massage today.
3. Explain how the term "scope of practice" applies to massage therapy.
4. Why does it seem so necessary to have rules, regulations, laws, and restrictions to govern the practice of massage?
5. Describe several reasons licenses may be revoked.
6. Explain the difference between a diploma, certification, and a license.
7. What is a code of ethics? Why is it important for a professional to commit to one in his or her practice?
8. Why do you think the items listed in the codes of ethics published by the AMTA (Fig. 2–1) and the NCBTMB (Appendix B) are so similar?
9. What are some of the common fears people have about working on the public? What are some of your fears? How can we get over fears about people?
10. Discuss a few of the human qualities needed to be a successful massage therapist.
11. Define the vocabulary terms at the beginning of this chapter.

3

EFFECTS AND BENEFITS
OF MASSAGE

*The student is to collect and evaluate facts. The facts are locked
up in the patient.*

Abraham Flexner

 LEARNING OBJECTIVES

After reading this chapter, students will be able to:
1. Discuss the healing mechanism of the body, including the Western mainstream medical approach and the Oriental approach.
2. Discuss the pain and inflammation processes, including the pain–spasm–pain cycle.
3. Describe how pain occurs in the body.
4. Describe how massage can help and hinder the inflammation process.
5. Discuss the physiological, psychological, and spiritual effects of massage.
6. Describe the effects of massage on various systems of the body.
7. Discuss massage movements used to effect changes in the various systems.
8. Identify the indications for massage.
9. Identify the conditions and reasons for *not* giving massage.
10. Identify conditions that are beyond their scope of practice, and understand that a referral to another health-related practitioner or doctor is needed.
11. Define the following vocabulary terms.

VOCABULARY TERMS

Contraindication	Indication	Nociceptor
Cycle of dependence	Inflammation	Pain–spasm–pain cycle
Endangerment site	Ischemia	Suppuration
Endorphin	Lymphocyte	Systemic condition
Exudate	Monocyte	
Homeostasis	Necrosis	

▪ INTRODUCTION

Why is it that, for centuries, men and women have touched and rubbed others to help them when they were in pain or injured? Why do so many people today seek professional massage to help them heal? Why does massage seem to relieve different ailments and injuries?

The answers to these questions and others relating massage to healing are at the heart of the profession today. Through understanding what massage does to the human being, we can decide how to massage in order to promote healing of a certain system or body part.

When a person visits a professional massage therapist, it is necessary to determine whether the conditions presented indicate massage. Massage therapists need to know when and why to treat, when and why not to treat, and when to refer a person to another healthcare practitioner. The body is a complex organism which reacts to massage in many ways. To understand the effects of massage, students must see the human being as a whole and, at the same time, as the sum of its various parts. For the purpose of this book, we will examine the benefits of massage on the physiological or body aspect of human beings, the psychological or mind aspect, and the metaphysical or emotional aspect. We will look at the methods by which the body heals and discuss how various cultures view the healing, pain, and inflammation processes.

▪ HEALING MECHANISMS OF THE BODY

Wellness Approach

Throughout our lives, our various components—body, mind, emotions, and spirit—try to stay in balance. This balance is both within ourselves (**homeostasis**) and with the environment in which we live. This is not an easy task, as everyone knows. Numerous books have been written on the myriad subjects entailed. However, we need to touch on a few of these subjects as we explore the changes that happen to us and the effect massage can have on these changes.

When homeostasis is not maintained within the body, an individual begins to feel disease, or not quite being him- or herself. Certain symptoms begin to manifest and the person may soon show outward signs that something is wrong. Help is usually sought at this point in the form of intervention. A medical doctor, homeopath, acupuncturist, or massage therapist may be seen for treatment. In mainstream Western medicine, the focus of attention is on disease. Getting rid of symptoms and chronic problems is the emphasis, not prevention or education towards holistic health. Seeing a doctor only when you are ill reinforces the belief that the doctor will heal you. Another belief by the medical profession is that human bodies are a mechanical set of parts. If something goes wrong, the philosophy is that you can get a new part. Seeing the body as a whole—with interrelated parts and as more than the sum of the parts—is needed to avoid this thinking. When prevention becomes the main focus and you see a healthcare practitioner for educational advice on what you can do for yourself, then the power to be healthy is returned to the individual.

Breaking this **cycle of dependence** on others for our balance of health is the focus of the holistic or alternative healthcare system. Taking control of maintaining or achieving good health and becoming educated on the subject can lead to a wellness program for ourselves. First, we need to educate ourselves on the various components of wellness: diet, exercise, relaxation techniques, positive thinking, anti-stress techniques or any other areas that you believe need to be investigated. Read books, talk to knowledgeable people in these fields, and then decide what actions are best for you to take.

Oriental Approach

In the Eastern model of wellness, health is not just the absence of illness but the entire balance of all things in your life. The mind–body connection is accepted and, in fact, the interactions among all parts of the human being are taken into consideration. This holistic view of the person sees the energy systems of the body controlling and directing the physical body (Fig. 3–1).

The energy system consists of a polarity of forces, *yin* and *yang*, that maintain balance (Fig. 3–2). The 6 yin and 6 yang channels together form an interior and exterior relationship in the body. The 12 channels represent the *meridian lines*. The energy flows along the channels or meridian lines that are connected to certain body organs. Disruptions in the flow of energy result in disease. Restoring the balance of energy restores health in the person and between the person and the rest of the world. A balanced lifestyle is necessary for a healthy human being. We will explain the Oriental approach in more detail in Chapter 8, when we discuss Oriental massage techniques.

What seems to be happening today in the Western world, especially in the massage profession, is a joining of these two models. In China today, these models for health have already merged. The Chinese patient can choose which type of medicine he or she prefers, Doctors of Traditional Chinese Medicine have also been trained in Western medical procedures. It may not be long before the medical professions in the West see the ancient traditions offering something that will enhance the Western medical model. Bill Moyers, in *Healing and the Mind* (1993), says, "Talking with different doctors during this journey, I realize that we do need a new

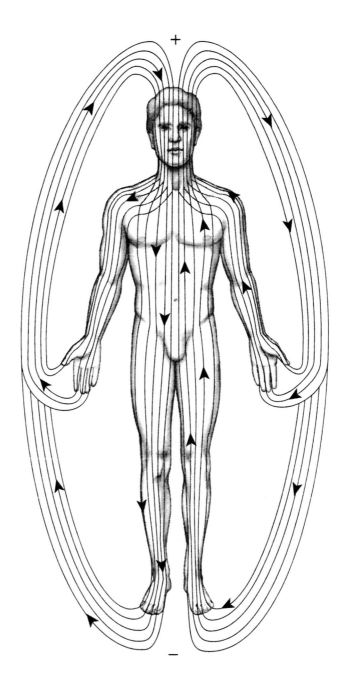

FIGURE 3–1. Energy systems.

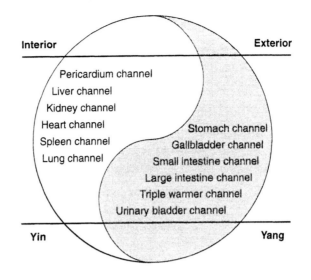

Interior   **Exterior**

Pericardium channel
Liver channel
Kidney channel
Heart channel   Stomach channel
Spleen channel   Gallbladder channel
Lung channel   Small intestine channel
                         Large intestine channel
                          Triple warmer channel
                       Urinary bladder channel

Yin   **Yang**

FIGURE 3–2. Yin/yang diagram.

medical paradigm that goes beyond 'body parts' medicine, and not only for the patients' sake." Seeing the person in a holistic manner could change the way we look at becoming whole.

▪ PAIN AND INFLAMMATION PROCESSES

Most people seek outside help because of pain. Yet the experience of pain is subjective, and each person's feeling of pain may be quite unique. The massage therapist's role is to offer a supportive and nonjudgmental presence.

Pain has physical, psychological, social, and financial components. It can be caused by physical ailments such as muscle spasm, insufficient blood flow to an area, or injured tissue. Mental or emotional states such as anguish, grief, indecision, anger, or fear may also cause pain. The client's emotional condition, past experiences with pain, learned behaviors, and cultural predisposition toward pain may also influence the client's experience with pain.

Physically, pain is caused by stimulation to nerve endings or receptors of pain, **nociceptors** found throughout the body in most tissues, somatic pain receptors in the skin and viscera for internal organs. When stimuli reach a certain level, called the *pain threshold*, the person feels the pain. Pain can be below the pain threshold, but then the person is not aware of it. Feeling pain is a defensive mechanism of the body, and when a client complains of pain, the therapist needs to evaluate the type of pain, its intensity, and its location. Anyone with an unexplained pain pattern should be referred to a physician. For example, continuous, increased, or severe pain must be evaluated by a physician.

Sources of Pain

Generally speaking, the sources of pain are divided into four categories. *Cutaneous pain* (from tissue damage) can be described as superficial, local, burning, sharp, and bright. *Somatic structures* like tendons, muscles, joints, and periosteum cause more diffuse pain that refers to other areas. *Functional or psychogenic pain* arises from emotions experienced as if from organic disorder. *Visceral pain* is often diffuse and results from strong abnormal distention, contractions, or ischemia of the gastrointestinal tract.

The body's reaction to pain minimizes tissue damage. Spinal cord reflexes help to remove painful body parts from the painful stimuli and the central nervous system reacts in a fight-or-flight response to pain. Pain travels up the spinal cord to the thalmus and cortex where it is modulated. Signals traveling down the spinal cord from the cerebellum can inhibit the pain signals at the spinal cord and decrease the level of pain felt.

Substances such as **endorphins,** released by the limbic system or brain stem, and enkephalin, produced by the hypothalmus, dorsal horns, and midbrain, are produced to moderate pain perception in the body. Norepinephrine, produced by the sympathetic nervous system, can also block pain.

Pain–Spasm–Pain Cycle

The **pain–spasm–pain cycle** is shown in Figure 3–3. This cycle of dysfunction—causing pain, voluntary splinting, in turn causing restricted movement, and resulting

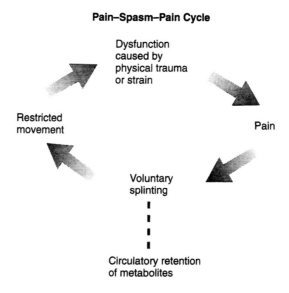

FIGURE 3–3. Pain–spasm–cycle: The cycle of dysfunction.

in more dysfunction—can become a vicious cycle and sometimes continues long after the original injury has healed. The massage therapist can intervene in the pain cycle by isolating the location and massaging the appropriate connective tissue and muscles. Often the touching and care given to a client by the massage therapist can interrupt the pain cycle long enough to allow tissue to begin healing. Naturally, if the skin is cut, massage is contraindicated. In that case, the therapist can reduce and sometimes alleviate the pain by working above and below the local area affected. Massage of the rest of the body may also be indicated.

Types of Pain

Muscle pain may start with a minor injury, muscle spasm, and impeded blood flow **(ischemia).** The muscle continues to contract, the blood supply is cut off, and toxins build up by excess energy burning. Now ischemic pain begins and general pain increases. Muscles continue to contract and restricted movement and dysfunction follows unless intervention occurs. Muscle pain can be described as sharp, aching, burning, or stabbing. When massage is applied to an area involved with the pain–spasm–pain cycle, the cycle may be broken. Pleasurable sensations from the therapist's touch and massage send messages to the brain that override the sensations of pain or distract the client from them. Pain will go down, its source separated from the ischemic tissue around it can be isolated, and spasms can be relieved. As a result of the massage, circulation increases: more oxygen and nutrients flood the area and irritants and toxins are removed from the area. Pain lessens and mobility of the area is increased.

Aching pain is constant pain caused by a visceral organ in trouble. Often this type of pain is removed from the location causing it and is called referred pain. For instance, back pain described as aching pain may be caused by visceral organs. Old injuries such as disc injuries in the back may also cause aching pain as time goes by. Such pain can be constant and often referred to other parts of the body. Reflexology may discern where this pain originates and what organ is in distress.

Deep pain often originates from deep inside the body, with the locality hard to pinpoint. It can become nauseating, and its effects on the autonomic system of the body are associated with sweating and raised blood pressure. Nearby muscles may become affected, as can tendons, bones, and ligaments. Continually spasming muscles cause pain; ischemia (heat and redness on the skin due to constricted blood flow in muscles) is present, and it further affects the muscle spasms and pain. A vicious cycle of pain–spasm–pain can occur.

Burning pain is hard to localize, lasts longer, and develops slowly. It often stimulates cardiac and respiratory activity. Burning pain may be described as feeling like a rope burn and is often caused by levels of fascia being stuck together.

Stabbing pain is short-lived, usually caused by cutting the skin or being jabbed by a sharp object. It is easily localized. (Again, massage is contraindicated if the skin is cut, but the therapist can sometimes work above and below the area.) Tendon tears or muscle tears may also cause stabbing pain at the time of injury. Fractures, too, cause this type of pain.

Inflammation

Inflammation is the body's attempt to fight infection or to cope with damage to body cells resulting from an injury. Disease-producing bacteria may enter the body, multiply, and harm cells. Healthy tissue may be destroyed, and when this occurs in a small area we consider it "local." When it spreads throughout the body, we consider it "systemic." A blow to the body, a sprain, excess heat or cold, or chemical exposure may also cause inflammation. The following symptoms of injury or infection are usually found in some degree: (1) pain, (2) redness, (3) swelling, (4) heat or fever, (5) loss of function, and eventually (6) formation of pus.

Inflammation may be acute, subacute, or chronic. An excess of fluid and cells is usually present or is issuing from the tissues (**exudate**) in an acute inflammation. When the vessel walls are affected, swelling (edema) and pain may occur. Exudates may be clear (serum) such as the discharge from a nasal cold; fibrinous, which causes adhesions to form as the tissues repair; bloody, as a result of small hemorrhages in the area; and purulent, due to bacteria. The formation of pus is called **suppuration.** The death of tissue, or **necrosis,** sometimes leaves an area that needs to be filled in with new tissue.

Massage is contraindicated in the presence of inflammation or any of the six symptoms mentioned earlier. Working above or below the affected area, however, will aid circulation, lymphatic flow, and overall healing. Naturally, anyone with a high fever (102°F or higher) or an inflammation lasting several days needs to be evaluated by a physician.

In longer inflammation situations, massage can increase the inflammation to speed up the process. By stimulating the lymphatic system as well, it can help the body produce more anti-inflammatory products. Working with the medical doctor in charge is essential for the best client care. Sometimes the body's reaction to the toxic substance or injury can cause a fever, which in itself may be enough to eliminate the invader, or cause the person to rest so that the body may begin to heal. The lymph system will carry the toxins to the lymph nodes, where they are destroyed by the white blood cells. An enlargement of lymph nodes during this time is not uncommon.

Pain and the inflammatory process are very complex. The massage therapist may be able to intervene in the pain process by giving a "careful" loving touch, thus changing the client's state of health. Over-the-counter pain killers are a multimillion dollar business in this country, and all of them create side effects in the body. Normally, massage does not create side effects and can intervene in the client's experience of pain and disease.

▪ PHYSIOLOGICAL EFFECTS OF MASSAGE

We can see from Box 3–1 that the physiological effects of massage are many and do indeed relate to the various systems of the body.

BOX 3-1   PHYSIOLOGICAL BENEFITS OF MASSAGE (EFFECTS ON THE BODY)

Improves circulation.

Relieves congestion.

Increases red blood cells temporarily.

Acts as a mechanical cleaner.

Increases lymph circulation.

Relaxes muscle spasms and helps prevent them.

Helps to prevent buildup of harmful fatigue products.

Improves muscle tone.

Compensates for lack of exercise.

Stimulates or sedates nervous system.

Aids temporary weight loss by helping absorption of fat (does not reduce fat cells).

Increases nutrition to tissues.

Increases excretion of fluids and waste products.

Encourages retention of certain elements such as nitrogen, phosphorus, and sulphur, which are necessary for tissue repair.

Helps reduce edema in the extremities.

Helps manage pain in labor and delivery and after accidents.

Reduces inflammation and swelling of joints.

Reduces pain.

Stretches connective tissue and helps minimize formation of adhesions and fibroses.

Improves circulation and nutrition of joints and hastens elimination of harmful deposits.

Improves digestion, metabolism, and assimilation.

Relieves scar tissue.

Reduces healing time.

Helps keep the skin healthy.

Circulatory System

Massage—and specifically Swedish massage—influences the circulatory system of the body. Upon massaging a particular body part, the blood rushes in, carrying increased oxygen and nutrients needed by the injured or stressed area. This increases venous flow of the blood back to the heart and lungs for reoxygenation and decreases venous pressure. Increased arterial circulation may result. Capillary pressure is thus reduced, and the fluid filtrating into extracellular space is decreased. Therefore, the load on the lymphatic system is reduced. This is accomplished through the pumping action of the heart and muscles. The congested area is nutritionally improved in the process and the congestion is lessened. The pumping action of compression and deep stroking during massage can increase the effectiveness of the massage. Even light stroking helps to dilate the capillaries so that blood flow may be increased.

Edema sometimes develops when the capillary pores become enlarged or capillary walls are destroyed and the capillary pressure increases. Then fluid movement from the capillary beds into interstitial space is increased. If the lymph flow is also obstructed, fluid collects most often in the ankles and hands. Prolonged standing can also increase gravity's effect on the extremities, as can extreme heat.

Because plasma proteins are needed to exert osmotic pressure to move fluids back into the capillaries from tissue spaces, the lack of them, as in starvation and malnutrition, creates edema. Liver disease may also affect this system by obstructing venous flow.

The severity of edema must be assessed by therapists to assure both the client and the therapist that massage may be performed. Pitting edema is assessed by applying digital pressure into the edemic site for several seconds. If an indentation occurs and remains after removal of the finger, massage is contraindicated.

Lymph and Lymphatic System

The lymph system is made up of one-way vein-like structures with loose flap-like valves that allow fluids from the tissue spaces to enter the capillaries. The collecting lymphatic structures continue to grow larger and eventually flow into one of two large lymph ducts and finally flow back into the blood. These tube-like vessels run from the extremities towards the heart. Fluid from the left side of the body and from the right side of the body below the chest area converges into the thoracic duct (left lymphatic duct). Lymph from the right side of the body, chest high, and the right arm flows into the right lymphatic duct (right thoracic duct). These two ducts enter the veins at the base of the neck where lymph mixes with blood plasma and becomes part of the general circulation.

But before the lymph reaches the veins, it passes through the nodes, where it travels through passages lined with cells that devour bacteria and where waste products and other foreign substances are filtered out. Unwanted substances are excreted. Thus, nodes help prevent the spread of disease to the entire body. They also manufacture **lymphocytes,** cells that fight disease and waste, and **monocytes**, large leukocytes, which have more protoplasm than lymphocytes, to add to the lymph transportation to the blood. Lymph nodes vary in size from very small to very large bean-shaped structures. The major areas for lymphatic nodes are the axilla, sternum, neck, and groin.

Massage encourages the lymphatic system's ability to clear away debris, fat, and unwanted substances. Passive joint movements will produce a similar pumping action across joints and will aid the lymphatic fluid to drain to other areas of the body where the fluid can be filtered in nearby lymph nodes (Fig. 3–4). Breathing seems to aid lymphatic draining in the thorax area. Massage strokes towards the heart also aid this process. In manual lymph drainage technique, the lymph is moved from distal to proximal areas. However, the proximal areas are generally cleared first. Strokes are light so as not to collapse the lymphatic system. General massage can greatly aid this system's function and also improve the body's immune

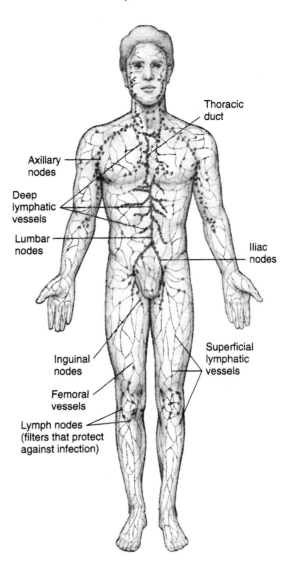

Thoracic
duct

Axillary
nodes

Deep
lymphatic
vessels

Lumbar
nodes

Iliac
nodes

Inguinal
nodes

Superficial
lymphatic
vessels

Femoral
vessels

Lymph nodes
(filters that protect
against infection)

FIGURE 3–4. Lymphatic drainage system.

system in the process. Manual lymphatic drainage is a well-known specialty in massage. Special training is needed to treat persons with postsurgery needs and other special lymphatic needs.

Nervous System

The nervous system can be stimulated or sedated by massage, depending on the type of massage given. Massage techniques that stimulate the nervous system include friction movements, percussion for a short time, and vibration. Sedative massage techniques include gentle gliding, light friction, and gentle kneading. Often a reflex effect occurs in which proprioceptors on the skin, being massaged, affect other areas of the body. For example, these include internal organs, vasomotor nerves, and areas in pain in other parts of the body.

When endorphins are released from the brain during massage, several responses may occur. Emotions are sometimes released, triggering memories of trauma stored both in the brain and in the tissues. The "fight-or-flight" response of the autonomic nervous system may be released. The parasympathetic system may also relax. Together, the parasympathetic and sympathetic systems work toward homeostasis. When an emotional and/or physiological state of trauma is reproduced for a client, responses similar to the original ones may occur. Old injuries can sometimes be reactivated in this way. Counseling is beyond the scope of a massage therapist's practice unless special training is received, but the massage therapist can often help the client to work through a session in which old emotions and injuries are relived. If the client needs additional help, a referral is indicated.

Respiratory System

Inhalation and exhalation of air in the respiratory system depend on the muscle system of the thorax, neck, abdominal region, pelvis, and legs. If any of these groups of muscles is not functioning fully, breathing is inhibited. Therefore, massage in these areas aids the functioning of muscles and breathing. Working with the breath during massage relaxes and aids the respiration as well as reduces pain.

Connective Tissue

The most abundant tissue in the body is connective tissue. It is most responsive to injury and/or trauma. Its function is to support, connect, and bind structures together. Layered in the body and surrounding all structures, connective tissue is kept in a semi-gelatinous state by a small electromagnetic (piezoelectric) current running through it. When connective tissue is injured or traumatized, the current lessens and the ground substance containing collagen, or matrix material, hardens. This causes hardening of the tissue and adhesion to nearby structures, immobilizing joints. Through massage, a softening can again occur. Space between the layers can be restored and joints can become mobile again. A spreading technique used in myofascial work, mechanical stretching and pulling of tissues, and compression and lifting tissue off the bones are all used to accomplish this. Connective tissue massage can be light work, as in cranial–sacral work, or it can be deep work aimed at joints, as in cross-fiber frictioning. Specialized training in myofascial and neuromuscular techniques will provide the massage student with advanced skills needed to work with accident and injury cases.

Massage is also helpful in cases of fractures that are healed, or in injury cases when sufficient time has passed and healing has taken place. Therapists working on a healthcare team in such cases will work with the physicians involved.

Excretory System

The excretory system of the body, like other systems, can become sluggish, out of balance, and blocked. Massage on the abdomen and lower back can, through reflex action, influence this system and bring it back into balance. Small gliding strokes, kneading, and friction can be used on the abdomen, while rocking and gentle vibration on the sacrum will also help. The direction of the strokes on the abdomen is clockwise due to the colon's position and process.

Muscular System

Muscles fatigued and sore from work can be revitalized through massage. Circulation through the muscles can be improved and thus tone can be enhanced, causing the muscles to be more firm and elastic. If muscles are too weak to function, they can be strengthened. Metabolically speaking, a muscle's chemical balance is maintained through regular activity. When overactivity or underactivity disrupts this balance, the massaged muscle may be urged back to normal. If injured, a muscle will heal more quickly with massage, as increased oxygen and nutrients are brought to the muscle with increased circulation. Muscles tightened and shortened often impair joint movement; massage can often improve mobility of joints. Passive range-of-motion movements before and after treatment will reveal the gains received from the massage. Active joint movements done by the client are similar to exercise and can strengthen and firm the muscles.

Energy Systems

The energy systems of the body have been identified since ancient times, yet modern medical research does not recognize such systems as "proven." However, many people realize several energy forces are at work within the human body. Given different names by various cultures—chi, ki, prana, auras, chakras, meridians—these systems can be enhanced and brought into balance by massage. Individual strokes and indeed, whole systems of massage have been developed to work primarily with energy systems. Among them are color therapy, aura stroking, polarity, and therapeutic touch. Caution is advised, however, that we substantiate our claims about what massage can do on these energy systems. An argument may be made that energy systems are not physical and should therefore be discussed under the psychological effects of massage (in the next section). Since physical energy can be felt, sometimes seen, and measured, I have chosen to discuss it here. If you feel more comfortable with it under the next heading, please feel free to move it for your own purposes.

■ PSYCHOLOGICAL EFFECTS OF MASSAGE

Much has been written and spoken about the body–mind connection in the past few years. Several recent books, TV shows, and interviews have investigated the role that the mind plays in influencing the body, and vice versa (see Box 3–2). The mind

BOX 3–2 PSYCHOLOGICAL BENEFITS OF MASSAGE (EFFECTS ON THE MIND)

Relieves stress, anxiety, and tension.
Makes a person feel marvelous.
Releases endorphins in the brain and promotes a natural "high" feeling.
Calms a hyperactive or agitated person.
Helps a person get in touch with his or her body.
Elevates the mood for a depressed or grieving person.
Activates the immune system towards healing.
Improves job performance.

is thought to influence us in deciding between disease and health. It can affect the immune system and sometimes influence decisions regarding life and death.

Hans Selye, the well-known author on stress, reminds us that the stress–pain–stress cycle is important in our lives today. When a person is under a lot of tension, body functions are affected. The fight-or-flight syndrome may be activated and the effects of other traumas and injuries can be accentuated. Many diseases are primarily, or secondarily, caused or exaggerated by stress. Stress lowers a person's pain threshold and various incidences that normally could be handled easily become monumental. Pain and additional stress often result. The person's reaction to stress and pain may be agitation or depression, depending upon the individual's emotional state. (See Chapter 10 for a more detailed discussion of stress and disease.)

Therefore, when massage is given and endorphins are released in the brain, the morphine-like chemicals act as pain reducers. This effect, coupled with the fact that someone who cares is tending to the client's needs, with the intention of healing, often has a positive effect on the client. Less pain is felt, stress and anxiety are lessened, and the client feels better. The pain threshold rises, and once again normal incidences are handled without adding more stress to the system or at least less pain is experienced. The person who has reacted to the stress–pain–stress cycle with withdrawal or depression symptoms begins to feel less depressed and more able to cope with life. If, after massage, a person feels less depressed and more in control of life, has a sense of well-being or just feels relaxed, massage has been helpful.

▪ EMOTIONAL AND SPIRITUAL EFFECTS OF MASSAGE

Many people believe that humans are more than just a compilation of parts and systems. Often that something extra has been linked to the heart or the emotional part of a human (see Box 3–3). Many psychologists today believe that therapy is enhanced by bodywork because of its ability to link the parts of us together. Certainly, massage affects the body and mind and, by alignment of various parts, puts us in touch with our cores, centers, or inner beings. Certain types of bodywork incorporate this idea in theory and practice (Rolfing®, SOMA, Neuromuscular Integration and Structural Alignment [NISA], CORE). Some believe this integration happens as

BOX 3–3   METAPHYSICAL BENEFITS OF MASSAGE (EFFECTS ON THE EMOTIONS)

Elevates the spirit.
Calms the worried mind.
Balances, integrates, and connects the whole being.
Puts the person in touch with self.
Helps create a state of heightened awareness or meditative state.
Shares intent to heal between client and therapist.
Brings hemispheres of brain together with core.

massage allows us a sense of heightened awareness or puts us into a meditative state. If we only call it the caring exchange between therapist and client, with the intent to heal, then something of the heart, mind, and hands has been exchanged.

▪ CURRENT RESEARCH

Current research on the effects of massage is being done in many places. Dr. Tiffany Field at the University of Miami School of Medicine's Touch Research Institute is conducting studies on infants, pregnant mothers, and geriatric patients. The John Fatzer Institute in Kalamazoo, Michigan, provided funding for the public television series "Healing and the Mind" with Bill Moyers. Dr. Bruce Pomeroy, University of Toronto, Canada, and Dr. Robert Becker have been doing research connected to massage for years. The Menninger Clinic in Topeka and Dr. Elmer Green have provided the validation of biofeedback. The newly formed American Massage Therapy Association (AMTA) Foundation is supporting several research projects each year. See Chapter 5 for more information.

These research projects, and many more, have provided us with information concerning massage's positive effect on anxiety and stress, its ability to influence the immune system, and its positive enhancement of adult job performance. Other research has shown that massage enhances the bonding between caregiver and abused, neglected children and improves poor sleep habits.

It is important that all aspects of people be kept in balance in research as well as in massage. It is only when we stay in balance within ourselves that we are the most effective therapists. As research on the total human being is completed, we can most effectively move massage to a higher professional standing among the medical and alternative therapies offered to the public.

▪ INDICATIONS FOR MASSAGE

Regaining health or attaining a new level of health is every person's desire. A condition in which massage is thought to help achieve these goals is called an **indication.**

Primary Benefits

For conditions related to mental fatigue, tension, stress, and insomnia, massage helps the client feel relaxed, more in control, less stressed, more confident, and more able to cope. Some of these changes are hard to measure, and are thought to be subjective, but are nevertheless real.

Various systems of the body such as the circulatory, lymphatic, and excretory systems are encouraged to return to their normal functions.

For muscle restrictions, fatigue, and related soft tissue damage as well as joint restrictions, massage helps the soft tissue and muscles to relax, tone, and return to normal functioning. This is done through improvement of circulation, removal of toxins, and the mechanical effect of stretching muscle fibers.

For headaches, pain, and irritated nerves such as in peripheral neuritis and sciatic pain, massage can soothe the nerves or excite them, depending on the type of massage given. Vibration, for example, is often done directly over the nerve path for nerve stimulation.

Skin function and tone can be improved. The provision of better circulation and nutrition to the skin through massage can assist in the prevention of blemishes.

After surgery, traumatized tissue can be helped to heal faster with reduced adhesions and less constriction through mechanical stretching, friction, and gentle gliding strokes. Edema can be lessened and blood circulation increased.

Secondary Benefits

In addition to the primary effects, massage can offer secondary aid to a person without treating the primary cause of his or her disease. Here are some examples:

- *Diabetes.* In persons with diabetes, massage often increases circulation, helping to prevent necrotic tissue formation in the legs and feet.
- *Immobility.* Persons who are immobile due to injury, wheelchair use, stroke, or cerebral palsy benefit from massage, which acts as mild exercise.
- *Weight management.* Persons on weight management programs can benefit from massage when the diet is combined with adequate exercise in a full program.
- *Degenerative conditions.* Persons with degenerative bone conditions find pain levels reduced and the health of the soft tissues maintained.
- *Inflammatory arthritis.* In persons with systemic conditions such as ankylosing spondylitis and rheumatoid arthritis, massage can help maintain mobility of joints and the health of the soft tissue when the client is in remission. Check with the client's physician to see if massage is indicated in a particular case.

Each case should be managed individually, depending on the health history, diagnosis, acuteness of stages, contraindications, and a physician's prescription or permission to treat.

▪ CONTRAINDICATIONS FOR MASSAGE

Massage cannot help every disease or injury. In some cases, massage can worsen the condition. In cases where massage cannot help the client and is not indicated, the condition or situation is called a **contraindication.** Sometimes a general or systemic condition dictates that the client cannot receive massage. However, if the condition is a local problem, massage may be given elsewhere on the body.

General or Systemic Conditions

Examples of general or **systemic conditions,** physiological conditions that affect the whole body, contraindicated for massage include fever, infectious disease, osteoporosis, pitting edema, kidney or heart disease, acute infections, phlebitis, thrombophlebitis, aneurysm, severe hematomas (especially cranial hematomas and malignancies), intoxication or drug use, psychosis, and the first 24 hours after scuba diving. In the last case, tiny nitrogen bubbles may go undetected and thus be a threat. Exceptions may be made in some of these conditions if the massage therapist is working on a medical team under the direction of a physician (for example, in the detoxification unit in a rehabilitative drug and alcohol facility). Refer to Box 3–4 for a case study.

Local Conditions

When massage is contraindicated by a local problem, it may be given elsewhere on the body. Examples of local contraindications include skin lesions, local edema, abdominal massage during pregnancy in the first trimester, varicose veins, and hernia.

Taking a complete health history at the first consultation with the client is essential. Then, if the massage therapist does not feel that massage can be done safely for any reason, a referral to a physician is indicated. Massage therapists do not diagnose. If diagnosis is needed, it should be done before massage is begun. If a client is already under a doctor's supervision or on medication, the massage therapist needs to contact the doctor and receive permission to treat that client.

 BOX 3–4   CASE STUDY

Susan, age 57, is referred by a physician after a recent mastectomy. The physician prescribes lymphatic drainage massage, range-of-motion movements, exercises, and general massage for stress reduction. Susan has received major surgery, is under a doctor's care, belongs to a cancer support group, and is seeing a psychotherapist for counseling. In this case, the massage therapist is clearly a valuable member of the healthcare team and should be in communication with each of the other practitioners involved. Together, they can provide her with the best of care.

A Reference Library

The massage therapist must know how to get information when it is needed. The following books are recommended for a start on a professional or reference library:

- *Taber's Encyclopedic Medical Dictionary*
- *The Physicians' Desk Reference* (medications & drugs)

No matter what the location is for your massage, you will always want to look up or follow up on health topics and medical terminology mentioned by your clients. (See Appendix F for a more complete listing.)

▪ SPECIAL POPULATIONS

Certain population groups receive massage regularly as part of their treatment. Babies, especially the premature (preemies), develop better and put on more weight when receiving daily touch and massage. Dr. Tiffany Field's research substantiates this. Through Seminar Network International School of Massage's outreach program, the critically ill and hospice patients receiving massage report comfort, pleasure, and relaxation. AIDS patients also report that caring touch is important to them. Some hospitals and programs, including psychiatric outpatient care and nursing homes, report beneficial results for their patients who receive massage. In these situations, many of us would say "the quality of life is what is important to us, not just the quantity."

In such cases, massage must be modified to suit the individual's need. Table massage, chair massage, light stroking, and holding a hand are all part of massage today. Strokes or touch need to be gentle, the length of treatment needs to be shortened, and the therapist needs to be nurturing in everything that he or she does.

▪ ENDANGERMENT SITES

Because of the possibility of damage to underlying tissues, vessels, nerves, and vital organs, massage therapists are cautioned to take special care when using direct pressure or deep manipulations in the following **endangerment sites** (see Fig. 3–5 to locate these sites).

1. Inferior to the ear, between ramus of mandible and occiput. Concern: styloid process, facial nerve, external carotid artery.
2. Anterior triangle of neck; medial line to sternocleidomastoid muscle. Concern: carotid artery, jugular vein, vagus nerve, and lymph nodes.
3. Posterior triangle of neck, sternocleidomastoid posterior to trapezius muscle including clavicle. Concern: brachial plexus nerves, brachiocephalic artery and vein, jugular vein and lymph nodes, subclavian arteries and veins.
4. Axilla, armpit. Concern: axillary artery and veins and nerves, cephalic vein, brachial plexus nerves, brachial artery.

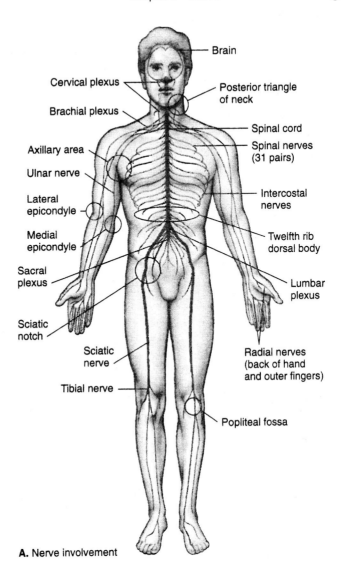

A. Nerve involvement

FIGURE 3–5. Endangerment sites. *(Continued)*

5. Medial brachium, upper inner arm between biceps and triceps. Concern: ulnar and median nerves, brachial artery, basilic vein and lymph nodes.
6. Sternal notch area of anterior throat. Concern: vessels and nerves to thyroid gland, including vagus nerve.
7. Medial and lateral epicondyle of humerus, elbow. Concern: ulnar and radial nerves.
8. Abdomen, umbilicus area, both sides, upper area under ribs. Concern: descending aorta and abdominal aorta.

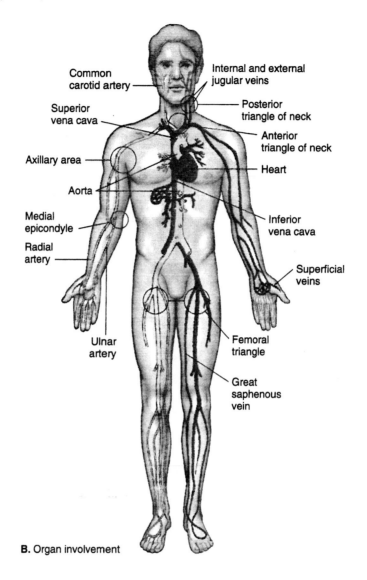

Common carotid artery

Internal and external jugular veins

Superior vena cava

Posterior triangle of neck

Anterior triangle of neck

Axillary area

Heart

Aorta

Medial epicondyle

Inferior vena cava

Radial artery

Superficial veins

Ulnar artery

Femoral triangle

Great saphenous vein

B. Organ involvement

FIGURE 3–5 (cont.). Endangerment sites.

9. Twelfth rib, upper lumbar area on dorsal surface. Concern: location of kidney and fragility of twelfth rib. Avoid heavy percussion.
10. Femoral triangle, anterior and medial upper leg including inguinal area. Concern: femoral artery, vein, and nerve; great saphoneous vein and lymph nodes; external iliac artery.
11. Sciatic notch. Concern: sciatic nerve.
12. Popliteal, fossa, posterior knee. Concern: tibial and peroneal nerve, popliteal artery and vein.

▪ REFERRALS

Often a massage therapist is called upon to refer a client to another healthcare practitioner or a physician for diagnosis and/or treatment (see Box 3–5). If a client seems ill or names a contraindication on the health history form, or if you observe in some way or intuit that something is beyond your scope of practice, the client needs to be referred to a professional whose training covers the specialty you deem necessary. "When in doubt, don't" is a good maxim covering the treatment of questionable conditions or symptoms for the massage therapist.

When other healthcare professionals send you clients, it is important to talk with them, the other professional about your mutual client, report back to them on progress, and even send them a thank-you card for the referral. In these ways, you serve your clients better and develop a working relationship with other healthcare professionals as well. It is a good idea to refer clients back to those who refer to you. You might even use the services yourself.

Students beginning professional massage careers are advised to become acquainted with other health-related professionals to whom they can refer clients. Many clients have their own primary physicians who will refer them to specialists. If not, a massage therapist can provide a list from which the client may choose. Those healthcare professionals most used include a primary MD, internist, neurologist, orthopedist, oncologist, podiatrist, psychotherapist, hypnotherapist, gynecologist, chiropractor, doctor of osteopathy, homeopathic physician, naturopath, and acupuncturist.

Once a client has been referred, he or she needs to bring back to you written documentation from the physician that indicates that massage may be performed. Never change or disregard doctor's orders without getting permission from her or

BOX 3–5   REFERRAL INDICATORS

Intuition.
Any changes in the skin, rashes, lumps, or nodes.
Persistent back pain.
Systemic conditions.
Infections or inflammation.
Bleeding or severe bruising.
Nausea, vomiting, or diarrhea.
Fever or a feeling of being very cold.
Extreme fatigue.
Pitting edema.
Severe mood changes, as in depression, grief, or anxiety.
Tingling in limbs.

him. For clarification, call the physician's office and ask the office manager or nurse for help. Keep any such documentation in the client's file.

Referral does not mean you have lost a client. Most of the time, the client will return for massage. Referrals are necessary for the client's safety as well as the therapist's safety. Always refer to another professional when anything signals the need to do so. Neither does referral mean that you cannot help your client on the day of his or her visit. Modalities such as polarity, therapeutic touch, and aura stroking can be done on anyone because touch is not required. The touch of your hand on someone's shoulder, a hug or firm handshake, and/or just listening intently to someone are always indicated in massage.

REVIEW QUESTIONS

1. Explain the way pain occurs.
2. Explain several ideas or components of both the mainstream medical approach in our society and the Oriental approach to wellness.
3. Discuss how you could be more responsible for your health, and how you could encourage your clients to do the same.
4. Discuss several different types of pain.
5. Describe how massage can both help and hinder the inflammation process.
6. The effects of massage were divided into three categories; what are they? Discuss the effects of massage on these three categories.
7. Name the systems of the body that massage affects.
8. Give an example of how the body can affect the mind. Give an example of how the mind can affect the body.
9. Describe how stress can affect the pain threshold.
10. Name a person doing current research on massage, and state how this research may help the profession.
11. Discuss the difference between the primary and secondary effects of massage.
12. Give examples of contraindications to massage and tell why.
13. Name and locate endangerment sites on the human body.
14. Give an example of a referral situation with a client.
15. Describe some of the conditions that indicate a referral.
16. How would you handle a client who refuses to see another healthcare professional?
17. Define the vocabulary terms at the beginning of this chapter.

SANITATION, SAFETY, AND PERSONAL HYGIENE

Nature, time, and patience are the three great physicians.

Proverbs

LEARNING OBJECTIVES

After reading this chapter, students will be able to:

1. Explain the importance of sanitation methods in massage.
2. Discuss the types of bacteria and viruses and their associated diseases.
3. Discuss sanitary conditions in the massage area concerning proper hand-washing techniques, sanitation of equipment, and use of disinfectants.
4. Prevent and control the spread of disease using sanitation procedures and safety means.
5. Explain safety procedures and practices in their professional businesses.
6. List good personal hygiene practices in a professional massage setting.
7. Define the following vocabulary terms.

VOCABULARY TERMS

Antiseptic	Bacilli	Disinfectant
Aseptic	Bacteria	Fission
Autoclave	Cocci	Fomite

Fumigant | Pathogen | Streptococci
Fungi | Protozoa | Vector
Metazoans | Rickettsiae | Virus
Microorganism | Spirilla
Parasite | Staphylococci

▪ INTRODUCTION

Many healthcare procedures today are considered common sense and taken for granted. Yet to remain healthy and prevent disease, care must be taken by everyone to maintain good sanitation practices and safety measures at all times. Infectious diseases are often transmitted by unclean hands, nails, and equipment. It is therefore imperative to have anything that touches the client impeccably clean. All linens, lubricants, therapist's hands, bathroom facilities, and any other equipment used in the massage must be clean at all times. The entire facility must also be clean, as this reflects the therapist's attitude toward cleanliness.

▪ MICROORGANISMS AND COMMON DISEASES

Microorganisms, like other living organisms, take in oxygen, use it for food energy, and excrete wastes. The total process is called metabolism. Microbes grow, reproduce, and die. Some can move under their own power; many can protect themselves by forming protective capsules or spores. Most are harmless to humans. Many, like yeast, are beneficial.

A few types of microbes are harmful to humans and causes disease. These are called **pathogens** (Box 4–1). An environment of warmth, darkness, moisture, and food as well as an oxygen supply aids their growth. Anaerobes (without oxygen) are one group of organisms that cause tetanus and gas gangrene. Aerobes (microbes that require oxygen to live) and facultative anaerobes (which live with or without oxygen) are others. The bacteria known as **staphylococci** and **streptococci** cause abscesses, pustules, boils, and blood poisoning. Warm temperature, moisture, and sometimes darkness can increase their growth.

Sunlight will sometimes destroy the bacteria. **Disinfectants** and **antiseptics,** chemical products that destroy the germ disease, slow their growth.

Five types of microorganisms exist: algae, fungi, bacteria, rickettsiae, and viruses.

Algae

Algae appear as green vegetation in ponds and, as far as we know, do not cause disease in humans.

Fungi

Including the molds and yeasts, **fungi** are commonly seen in kitchens as the fuzzy patches found on fruit, the greenish growth on old bread, and the blue veins in some

BOX 4–1   COMMON TYPES OF PATHOGENIC ORGANISMS

Bacteria: three forms (spherical, rod-shaped, spiral); minute unicellular microorganisms that secrete toxic substances into human cells and can produce resistant forms that become difficult to destroy.

Fungi: plant-like organisms; single cells like yeasts or filament as in molds.

Viruses: microscopic, parasitic agents that transmit disease by invading host cells.

Protozoa and pathogenic animals: **protozoa** are simple, single-celled organisms; **metazoans** are members of the primary division in the animal kingdom whose cells have outer and inner walls, including all animals higher than protozoans.

Rickettsiae: the microorganisms parasitic in ticks and lice transmissible to animals and humans.

---

cheeses. Molds spread through the air, depositing spores on multiple surfaces. Ringworm and athlete's foot are common fungal diseases. Yeasts spread by producing a bud and spreading out. Thrush, or moniliasis, is caused by a pathogenic yeast.

Bacteria

Bacteria are unicellular organisms having both animal and plant characteristics. Bacteria are also known as germs or microbes. Single-celled organisms, pathogenic bacteria are divided into three groups—cocci, bacilli, and spirilla (see Fig. 4–1).

- **Cocci** are spherical and responsible for abscesses, blood poisoning, and pneumonia.
- **Bacilli** are rod-shaped and responsible for typhoid fever, tuberculosis, lock jaw, and diphtheria.
- **Spirilla** are curved or spiral-shaped and responsible for syphilis.

Bacteria grow by dividing into two; this is called **fission.** Some develop a spore capsule when conditions are unfavorable and can be inactive for a time. These bacteria are difficult to control and destroy.

All pathogens are killed at 100°C (212°F), except the spore formers. Steam under pressure is the known destroyer. An **autoclave,** a dry heat cabinet used to sanitize objects, is used in hospitals to destroy all bacteria.

Staphylococci are normal inhabitants on the human skin, but can kill when they causes serious infections, especially in infants or after surgery. Streptococci are present in a healthy respiratory system, but cause "strep throat" when they cause disease.

Other bacteria include *Pseudomonas,* which causes pus-forming infections; *Salmonella,* which causes intestinal infections; and *Clostridium,* difficult to kill, which causes gas gangrene and botulism.

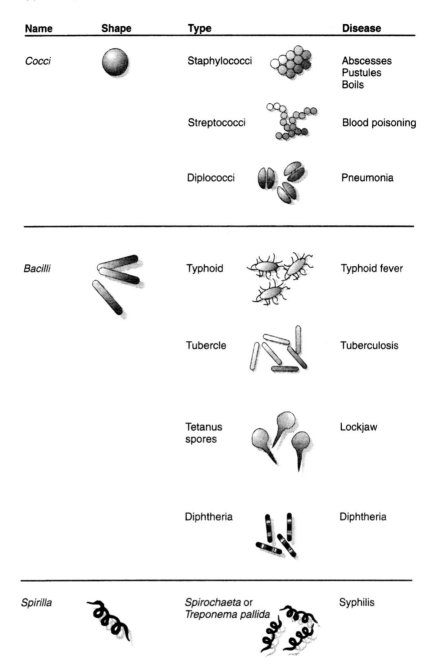

Name	Shape	Type		Disease
Cocci		Staphylococci		Abscesses Pustules Boils
		Streptococci		Blood poisoning
		Diplococci		Pneumonia
Bacilli		Typhoid		Typhoid fever
		Tubercle		Tuberculosis
		Tetanus spores		Lockjaw
		Diphtheria		Diphtheria
Spirilla		*Spirochaeta* or *Treponema pallida*		Syphilis

FIGURE 4–1. Harmful bacteria include cocci, bacilli, and spirilla.

Rickettsiae

Rickettsiae are microorganisms which are parasitic in ticks and lice and are transmissible to other animals and man. Typhus is an example of a transmitted disease to man. **Parasites** are organisms that live within, on, or at the expense of another. Rickettsiae can grow only in living tissue within the host cells. They are transmitted by carrier insects through a bite. They are readily killed by heat.

Viruses

Viruses, parasitic pathogen agents that trasmit disease, have no means of locomotion, no source of power, and no ability to grow. Viruses reproduce only when they invade a living cell. Most methods of destroying viruses are not very satisfactory, nor are drugs very effective for control. Vaccination helps in the prevention of smallpox, measles, and polio.

Contagion

Many diseases are contagious, that is, communicable and spread by contact, either indirect contact or through the air. **Fomites** are nonliving carriers of pathogens, which include water, air, food, dust, and soil. **Vectors** are living carriers of disease such as rats, fleas, and lice.

The chain needed for the spread of disease depends on (1) a susceptible host, (2) a portal of entry into the human body, (3) the presence of organisms of disease, (4) a reservoir for the organisms, and (5) a portal of exit for transmission of the organism.

The best way to assure the disease cannot use this chain is to use **aseptic** (germ-free) techniques whenever possible.

The best way to protect oneself as a massage therapist is not to work on people who are ill or have a contagious disease. Nor should the therapist work on clients when he or she is diseased. Any open wound or infection on the exposed body or any contagious disease is a contraindication to massage. Keeping oneself and one's surroundings clean and sanitary is the best precaution against disease.

▪ SANITATION PRACTICES

The key to the prevention of pathogenic organisms entering the skin is to maintain sanitary conditions. This includes paying attention to air quality, sanitizing surfaces and containers in the laundry of linens, cleaning linens for every client, and washing the hands before and after every client with antibacterial or fungicidal soap (see Box 4–2).

The following general sanitary practices are recommended in a massage practice:

1. Store linens away from personal effects and clothing. Clean linens should be separated from unsanitized or used linens. If used linens are stored in hampers or receptacles, they should be covered. Clean linens can be stored

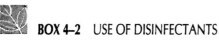

BOX 4–2   USE OF DISINFECTANTS

- *Ethyl or grain alcohol.* Use a 70 percent solution to rinse hands, tops of massage tables, and implements.
- *Formalin.* Use as an antiseptic or disinfectant. A 25 percent solution is used to immerse brushes and other implements. Time: 10 minutes.
- *Quaternary ammonium compounds.* Tablet or liquid. Disinfectant for a short time. Immerse 1 to 5 minutes in a 1:1,000 solution. Nontoxic, odorless, colorless, and stable. Good for spatulas, nail clippers, and other implements.
- *Lysol or creosol.* A 5 to 10 percent solution is good for floors, restrooms, countertops.

---

on shelves or in closed cabinets. Neither should be left open to the air. Bleach should be used along with hot water for washing used linens.

2. Never practice massage if you are infected with any communicable disease or if you have an infected or open wound.
3. Sanitize any aids used in massage—such as loofas, spatulas, T-bars, mechanical aids, nail clippers, and brushes—before each use. The disinfectant container should be large enough so that an object can be immersed in it after the object has been washed in hot water and soap. A dry or cabinet sanitizer using an active **fumigant,** a chemical used to disinfect a room, is another choice. Boiling objects at 212°F (100°C) for 20 minutes is another suggestion. An autoclave is sometimes used in the medical field.
4. Wash your hands and arms (if used in therapy) before every client. This is the best way to avoid pathogens entering the skin. Use antibacterial or antifungal soap and use paper toweling to dry the skin. In places where bathrooms are not convenient (sporting events, malls), an alcohol wash is the substitute. Normally, use hot water and create a good lather with soap and work it between fingers and under nails. Rinse in hot water and dry with paper towels. You can use the drying towel to turn off the tap and open the door.
5. When filling your lubricant container from a larger bulk container, be careful not to touch the lubricant. Unused lubricant coming into contact with your hands or another surface should be discarded.
6. Keep your massage tables clean and in good repair. Clean after each client with soap and water, 10 percent bleach, and/or wipe down with alcohol.
7. Keep supplies organized and properly labeled, with tops secure and clean.
8. Use a spatula, not your fingers, to remove a product from its container.
9. Wash your linens as quickly as you can after use. Oils are often hard to remove from linens, especially after long use. There are commercial products

on the market just for this purpose, but often a small quantity of Spic and Span or dishwasher detergent such as Cascade added to the laundry soap will do the job as well.

10. Remember, the entire facility where you practice massage reflects your cleanliness habits as well as your atmosphere for massage. Check equipment often for safety. Consider a policy against using lighted incense and candles. Have a first-aid kit; keep it current and always in the same place for easy access. Have heating and cooling systems checked regularly and change the filters often. Keep walkways clear and well lighted.

11. Keep the surfaces and floors clean throughout your facility. Sanitize bathrooms and surfaces that come in contact with clients.

▪ SPECIAL CONDITIONS FOR MASSAGE THERAPISTS

Under normal conditions in a massage practice, the therapist is under no risk when sanitary conditions are maintained, either in the contact with a client or in the follow-up cleaning of linens or treatment room. Occasionally, however, extra precautions need to be taken.

For instance, menstrual blood may leak onto the table. Lymphatic drainage often produces excess liquid drained from the body. Urine or feces can leak from the body onto linens, as can vomit. Any heavy massage or bodywork may trigger leakage of body fluids from the client. When this situation occurs, extra care needs to be administered in the cleanup process and in the handling and washing of linens.

In any of the cases mentioned, the therapist needs to wear single-use disposable latex gloves. (Generally, gloves marked "vinyl" are not safe.) To clean up a fluid "spill," use a 10 percent bleach solution on the area, working towards the center of the spill so as to prevent spreading of the contaminant. Wash the massage table with a strong disinfectant and let it air dry. If your skin comes into contact with body fluids, wash the body part thoroughly with an antiviral agent such as the 10 percent bleach solution. Hot, soapy water will kill most viruses.

If linens have been contaminated, care is needed in transferring them to the laundry area. Carefully ball up the linens with the "spill" area to the inside. Use gloves in carrying them and transport in a disposable plastic bag. Do not put with other linens waiting to be laundered. Use a strong bleach solution when washing these linens.

Remember, massage therapists want to protect themselves and their clients at the same time. If clients are in an immune-suppressed state, they must be protected from germs, too.

If you are working with patients with communicable diseases in a hospital or clinic, you are probably following medical procedures in dealing with them. If you have questions about what procedures to follow in your situation, contact the Centers for Disease Control and Prevention at (404) 332-4555 or at (888) 329-4232 (toll-free).

▪ SAFETY PRACTICES AND ACCIDENT PREVENTION

No matter where one works, safety practices are needed for both the client's and therapist's benefit. Like sanitation, safety practices protect both the client and the therapist from harm and should be followed every day. With many things, prevention is the best policy.

For fire safety, know the location of fire extinguishers in your building and how to use them. Exit signs should be well lit and easy to see. Know an evacuation route from your building. Emergency numbers should be posted by every telephone. Check all electric cords regularly and keep all equipment in good repair.

Take the following steps to help prevent accidents:

- Ask any association of persons with disabilities what help is needed and follow their instructions.
- Use good lighting in all rooms.
- Keep walkways and outside entrances clear and uncluttered.
- Keep current on your cardiopulmonary resuscitation (CPR) and first-aid certifications.
- Do not leave the elderly, infants, young children, handicapped persons, or third-trimester pregnancy clients alone. They may need help.
- Check with clients before using new products. They may be sensitive or allergic to them.
- Use proper body mechanics when lifting or helping clients and when performing your massage. This protects you from injury.
- Only work within your scope of practice and "do no harm."

▪ PERSONAL HYGIENE

To promote ourselves as massage therapists and to exhibit professionalism, we need to promote our own health. A healthy body, mind, and spirit does not get ill often. If we are healthy, our clients will listen to us when we speak about health. In any personal service business, good grooming is also very important. It portrays someone who cares about himself or herself as well as about clients.

Several areas regarding personal health and hygiene need to be reviewed. They are as follows:

1. Do not smoke. Smoking is known to cause health problems in both smokers and nonsmokers. Many people are sensitive or allergic to smoke, and others find the lingering odor obnoxious. If you do smoke, keep the massage room smoke-free and smoke outside the building during business hours. Clean your breath and mouth immediately after smoking. Change clothes often and wash your hair often.
2. Adhere to personal hygiene habits faithfully: daily baths or showers, clean hair and nails, use of deodorant as needed, avoidance of bad breath, and clean clothes. Hair should be neat and away from the face. It should be pinned up if it is long. Your hair should not touch the client during a

massage. Remove all jewelry. If you perspire heavily, wear head and wrist sweat bands to avoid perspiring on the client.

A uniform is not necessary, however, your clothing should be loose fitting but should not drag on the client during the massage. Choose clothing that breathes and keeps you cool while working. If you do choose a uniform, remember to think about frequent laundering and oil stains. Shoes should be comfortable and clean, free from dirt and stains.

3. Build personal free time into your schedule. Take time for stress-free activities and exercise. Burn out among massage therapists is high. Take care of your arms and hands. Get massage regularly. If you don't get bodywork weekly, how can you expect your clients to do it? You need to continuously work on improving your health if you want your clients to take you seriously and do the same.

4. Do not use drugs or alcohol in your place of business. Drugs and alcohol affect thinking processes and decision making. The body is toxic and tired after consumption and clients need you at your best.

In thinking about any health-related subject you might be discussing with a client, the motto is: "Do as I do, not as I say."

Remember, if either therapist or client has a contagious disease or a contraindication for massage, do not do massage or bodywork on the client. Refer the client to the proper healthcare practitioner or physician, or home if the condition is a minor cold or flu. You can reschedule the appointment at another time.

REVIEW QUESTIONS

1. Why is it important to maintain sanitary conditions in your massage practice?
2. Explain conditions that cause disease most of the time.
3. Explain proper handwashing techniques, ways of sanitizing equipment, and the proper use of disinfectants.
4. Describe the four types of pathogenic organisms.
5. Name some of the diseases caused by each of the four types of pathogenic organisms.
6. Discuss the general sanitation practices recommended.
7. Describe the use of disinfectants in regard to massage tables, bathrooms, counters, and massage implements.
8. Describe extra precautions that the therapist needs to take when the client's body fluids have escaped.
9. Discuss safety practices in regard to fire safety, preventing accidents, and personal hygiene.

10. Discuss personal hygiene practices that therapists need to follow with regard to their clients.
11. Discuss personal practices that therapists need to follow regarding their own health.
12. What can you do if a client shows up with symptoms or signs of a contagious disease?
13. Define the vocabulary terms at the beginning of this chapter.

THE SCIENCE AND ART OF MASSAGE

Health is not a condition of matter, but of mind; nor can the material senses bear reliable testimony on the subject of health.

Mary Baker Eddy

LEARNING OBJECTIVES

After reading this chapter, students will be able to:
1. Discuss the role of the mind and how it interacts with the body.
2. Explain why it is so difficult to study humans in their wholeness.
3. Explain the mainstream medical approach and how it is working today in the massage profession.
4. List several modalities that are classifed as energetic approaches.
5. Discuss several things to look for in postural assessment/body reading.
6. Describe several current research projects.
7. Define the following vocabulary terms.

VOCABULARY TERMS

Anatomy
Cranial–sacral technique
Cryotherapy
Energetic approach
Fibromyalgia

Lymphatic massage
Mainstream medical
   approach
Myofascial pain
Physiology

Postural assess-
   ment/body
   reading
Psychoneuroim-
   munology

▪ INTRODUCTION

Many people today, inside and outside the medical field, recognize that the mind and body make up a unit. Experienced massage therapists realize they are often dealing with more than sore neck muscles or a painful low back in a client. Because of recent research in the medical world, a new branch of medical science has come into being, **psychoneuroimmunology** (*psycho* for mind, *neuro* for the neuroendocrine system, and *immunology* for the immune system); this new branch of medical science seeks to understand how the various parts of humans are put together and how they operate.

As far back as the classical Greek period, historians have made reference to the various components of humans. Even before that, the esoteric communities were operating under the premise that people lived and worked in a world both physical and unseen. The split between the mind and body is not new. What is new is the acceptance by a major portion of the medical profession of the fact that we are more than flesh and bones and the desire to explore and try to understand how all the parts work together and influence each other. Without going into various religious thoughts (that are beyond the scope of this book), let us think of the body as the physical aspects, the flesh and bones; the emotions as the feelings a person has and expresses; the mind as the operator of the brain and the body; the spirit as the underlying force that governs and directs the whole.

Every human being is unique. Each person will experience injury, pain, illness, or degree of health differently and will view them differently. We have to consider the whole person when we deal with others in our practices.

▪ BODY, MIND, SPIRIT CONNECTION

Specialization in every aspect of life divides subjects and people into parts in order to study them. In fact, this division is necessary in studying **anatomy,** the structure of the body, and **physiology,** how they function together. Anatomy and physiology are the basis of the Western philosophy of medicine. Yet, when we treat people, we too often separate the feelings or thoughts from the disease of the body. We think we know more about the body than about the mind or spirit, so we often treat the body first. There is perhaps reason or understanding for this if we look at the various parts of humans and what is revealed to us in physical form. Yet, we know that any one part affects the whole. The body can affect the emotions. The visceral organs can affect the mind. The spirit can affect the body. As Dr. David Felten says in *Healing and the Mind:*

> *Now there is overwhelming evidence that hormones and neurotransmitters can influence the activities of the immune system and that products of the immune system can influence the brain (Moyers, p. 213).*

Dr. Dean Ornish adds:

> *As physicians, we can deliberately or inadvertently increase the negative effects of the mind on the body—but we can also use the mind to have a healing effect on the heart (Moyers, p. 93).*

Look at Figure 5–1 for a moment. A human being is a unit. The body, emotions, mind, and spirit are each a unit of energy within a whole unit of energy. Matter is energy, as Einstein taught us. When energy is focused on any part of the whole, matter or energy moves and changes occur in the other units. For example, a person can become so angry over an incident that he or she cannot stop thinking about it and discussing it over and over with anyone who will listen. The mind–body focuses on anger. The feelings are of hate and revenge. Soon the stomach starts to sour and indigestion and pain occur. As time goes on, the spirit of the person may become disheartened and diverted from its natural course. Violence and death may be the outcome if this pattern is not broken or reversed.

If we turn this energy around and direct a person's mind, emotions, spirit, and body towards healing and health, then we find things happening like spontaneous remissions, "miraculous" healings, and longer lives than expected. We find the quality of their lives has been improved as well. How well we live is perhaps more

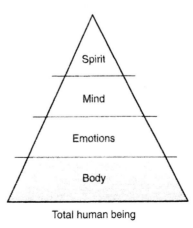

Total human being

FIGURE 5–1. Total human being.

important than how long we live. "It's important to give life to years, not just years to life" (Moyers, 1993, p. 41).

Several tenets of belief about dealing with the whole person come to mind:

1. It is important to treat the whole person.
2. The patient is his or her own healer.
3. How the therapist thinks is very important to the client's improvement and health.
4. The confidence clients have in the therapy, the therapist, and in themselves is very important to healing and must not be broken.

▪ THE MAINSTREAM APPROACH

This focus on the whole person becomes crucial when we explore the medical model of massage theory and practice. Throughout history, some aspect of massage has often been a part of medicine. Today, in Europe and China, massage and hydrotherapy techniques merge into hospital care, sometimes being performed by physicians themselves and often given by other specialized, trained personnel. In the United States and Canada, massage therapists enter hospitals and clinics every day, giving massage to infants and new mothers, manual lymphatic drainage to postsurgery patients, and seated massage to family members of patients as well as hospital staff. To work in a professional and clinical setting, massage therapists need to be trained in medical terminology, professional behavior, hospital and clinic protocol, pathological conditions, and anatomy and physiology. This scenario of training and practice is thought of as the **mainstream medical approach** of massage. Of course, it is not the only scenario in massage, nor is it the most popular or the most frequent. The Canadian provinces of British Columbia and Ontario prepare their students over their 2- to 3-year courses for the mainstream medical approach to practice.

Even in this setting, as massage therapists, we need to find ways to show our care and good touch. Dr. Ron Anderson, of Parkland hospital in Dallas, talks in *Healing and the Mind* about this way of wholeness and caring:

> *The attitude of caring has always been a part of the human being's experience. We just forget it at times of war, in high tech–high stress situations, and at moments of selfishness when talking seems better than listening. Yet it has never been as important to people's health and fulfillment as it is right now (Moyers, 1993).*

Some people believe that the emotions may be the link between the body and the mind. Dr. Candace Pert, Professor at the Center for Molecular and Behavior Neuroscience, thinks so. "Emotions might actually be the link between the mind and the body." When Bill Moyers asks her: "What's down there?" (in the body), she answers:

> *Peptides, receptors, cells. The receptors are dynamic. They're wiggling, vibrating energy molecules that are not only changing their shape from millisecond to millisecond,*

but actually changing what they're coupled to. One moment they're coupled up to one protein in the membrane, and the next moment they can couple up to another. It's a very dynamic, fluid system (Moyers, 1993, p. 186).

Moyers then asks: "Are you saying that we're just a circuit of chemicals?"
Dr. Pert replies:

Well, that gets to be a philosophical question. One way to phrase it would be, can we account for all human phenomena in terms of chemicals? I personally think there are many phenomena that we can't explain without going into energy. As a scientist, I believe that we're going to understand everything one day, but that this understanding will require bringing in a realm we don't understand at all yet. We're going to have to bring in that extra-energy realm, the realm of spirit and soul that Descartes kicked out of Western scientific thought (Moyers, 1993, p. 186).

Certainly, experienced massage therapists can tell you about countless instances when bodywork has elicited a memory or emotions from the past. Clients often tell of past injuries, accidents, or abuse that they have experienced. Somatic Release has become a popular modality today as therapists realize that they need specialized training in helping their clients handle and work through their responses to their treatments.

I had a lovely 80-year-old client, Viola, who loved the color purple. She told and retold the story of getting a vaccination on her upper left thigh at age 5. She never talked about this incident unless I was massaging that leg at exactly the spot where the scar occurred. She had no pain there, but massaging the spot brought back to her the same story each time a massage was given.

▪ THE ENERGETIC APPROACH OR MODEL

Another model in massage today is the **energetic approach.** It is based on either Chinese or ancient Indian Ayurvedic theory. Its prime objective is holistic health. There are many kinds of energetic treatments and they are not always hands-on. For example, the treatments of Amma and Hoshino are hands-on body treatments, while chakra balancing, as in polarity, may be done with a hands-on method or with hands held slightly off the body. Thai massage involves both hands-on massage and joint stretching as well as clearing the body along the meridian lines. Color therapy is often done with light aimed at the body from a prism machine, and healing through the human energy field may or may not involve actual hands-on treatment. Therapeutic touch is done 3 to 4 inches off the body. No matter how these various therapies are performed, the basis of how the body works in the energetic model is ancient. Body functions relating to how energy (chi or qi) is flowing or balanced throughout the body is the central concept. There are other concepts which are important (Sohn, 1988). Figure 5–2 shows the use of energy in the therapist as he or she is massaging.

If the mind–body relationship is one and the same thing, as many believe, then the energy force of the mind–brain is interchangeable with the energy force of

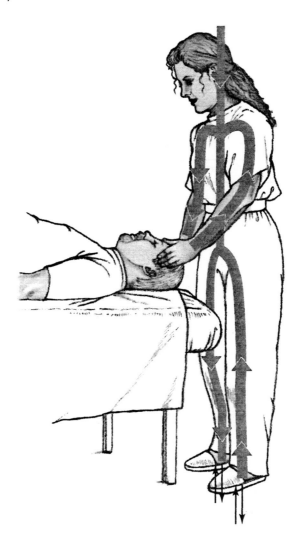

FIGURE 5–2. Use of therapist's energy during a massage. The therapist's body is used as a conduit. The right side of the body transmits positive energy to the client, while the left side receives negative energy, to be released.

the body. The entire body may be one large energy system with the interplay of structure, function, and energy flow. This idea is not new, but it may help us to see that the mainstream medical approach and the energetic approach can complement each other. The Western and Eastern cultures may be merging in medicine as medical doctors like Dr. David Eisenberg travel to China to study and understand Traditional Chinese Medicine (TCM) and how it might interact with Western medicine (Moyers, 1993).

▪ MAINSTREAM MEDICAL APPROACH AND ENERGETIC APPROACH

The mainstream medical approach, massage theory and practice directed toward the medical fields, and energetic approach or, healing and massage using energy techniques, are but two popular models used today in the massage field. It is not important which model we choose but it is very important that common threads exist in whatever model we choose. The mind/body/emotions/spirit or wholeness concept transcends any model. The underlying relationship with the client allows the therapist to know what the client expects and what he or she wants. Until we know that and blend it with our ideas of what should be offered in the treatment, we do not have a treatment plan that will work. Massage, like the rest of life, needs to be a win–win situation between the therapist and the client. It doesn't matter how competent we are at massage if we do not satisfy our clients in the process. Being competent and satisfying our clients' needs is the ultimate scenario.

▪ POSTURAL ASSESSMENT/BODY READING

It has long been thought that the body we see is more than the sum of all of its parts. **Postural assessment/body reading** means to understand what the body is telling us. The therapist sees visual clues that can reveal not only differences in body symmetry but also our clients' thoughts, feelings, behavior, and past experiences. This information can be used by the massage therapist to relieve those patterns, release tissue and emotions, change the client's thinking, and mold him or her into a free personality.

The body is a roadmap of our lives. It can be read to see where underdevelopment or overdevelopment has taken place. It reveals areas of stagnant energy, or leaks and holes in the energy pattern. It can tell you where areas have been compromised and compensations have developed. It can allow you to see emotional attitudes as well as fears and rejections.

It takes time to develop both "hard seeing" of the outer and blatant issues as well as "soft seeing," seeing the inside of the person.

Hard seeing has to do with seeing postural, skin, and structural conditions of the client. By looking at body parts, balance in the system, relationships of extremities to related joints, and dominance of one side of the body, you can begin to see how the body has adjusted to life's experiences. Hard seeing is a function of the left hemisphere of the brain. Keep your eyes opened and focused and look hard to see minute and subtle differences in the physical body.

Soft seeing has to do with seeing inside the client. How have the client's adaptations affected the inner being? Is the core strong or weakened? Is the spirit vital or subdued? Has the vitality or energy been compromised, or can this person regain his or her health? Soft seeing is a function of the right hemisphere of the brain. Keep your eyes half closed, and softly focused, to see the inner being and make contact with it.

Postural assessment/body reading does not imply judgment. It is important that as therapists we do not label our clients, or impose conditions upon them. We will bypass these pitfalls by approaching our clients from our hearts and making contact with theirs. By asking for information to verify our reading of the body and getting confirmation of our inferences, we can avoid much of the subjectiveness that science scorns.

The more you practice using your intuition, the more you will, in time, be able to see the whole being standing before you (Box 5–1).

Generally speaking, where you see a problem area, ask yourself the function of that body part. An example might be a problem with one of the senses (eyes, ears, nose, or throat). Ask yourself why this person is having difficulties with seeing, hearing, smelling, or talking. The cause of the problem will lie in the body part. If the body part is an organ, then look to the function and the systemic connection to the whole person. Sometimes, too, the chakra and its energy function can tell you what is wrong.

Although modern medicine does not recognize this method of observation, the psychological field does. Reich, Lowen, and Pirerkos all have written about body language.

When dealing with a client and doing body reading, always confirm your observations with the client. In this manner, the information exchanged can be a part of your clinical notes (SOAP notes).

▪ CURRENT RESEARCH

The *Bodywork Knowledge Base* collected by Richard Van Why (1991) is an enlightening survey of research involving massage from 1965 to 1989. Subjects include athletic massage; **lymphatic massage** which aids the body to balance the lymphatic system; pain management; and **myofascial pain syndrome** caused by the hardening of fascia and muscles. Also discussed are vibration therapy in children with cerebral palsy; treatment of **fibromyalgia** (inflammation of connective tissue); pain reduction; massage and the knee; treatment of soft tissue after spinal injury; muscle pain syndromes; **cryotherapy** (the use of ice in therapy); massage for newborns; **cranial–sacral** findings (manipulation of cranial and sacral fluid systems and skull bones); and developmental problems in children.

Current research is proving to the medical field as well as to the public that massage can be a much more useful tool in our health kit than most people previously thought. A few of the current research projects deserve our attention.

At the University of Miami Medical School's Touch Research Institute, Dr. Tiffany Field has been working on showing the effects of touch and stroking massage on the growth and development of infants, on pregnant mothers, and on geriatric patients. The Touch Institute was established in 1992 and is the only center in the world devoted solely to the study of touch and its application in science and medicine. Research under the direction of Dr. Field has shown that touch therapy has numerous beneficial effects on human well-being. "Specifically, we have shown that massage can induce weight gain in premature infants, alleviates depressive symptoms, reduces stress hormones, alleviates pain and positively alters the immune system in children and adults with various medical conditions" (Field, 1997).

BOX 5-1 THINGS TO LOOK FOR IN A CLIENT

- Differences in size, shape, and texture from one body part to another.
- The focus of energy in the body.
- Splits from side to side, top to bottom, back to front. Energy and vitality, size, and shape may differ. Figure 5–3A shows shoulder differences. Overbalance and underbalance is another way to look at splits.
- Balance, support, or lack of it in legs and feet. They support us and take us where we want to go in life. Insecurity is often expressed in our legs and feet.
- Pelvis movement or lack of it in a person's gait. Is there a pelvis tilt anterior or posterior? Stability, security, and sexual tension are often seen in the pelvis.
- Areas of boundaries between parts such as the chest and abdomen. Areas such as these should be integrated, not cut off. Fear is often expressed on boundary lines. Armoring sometimes occurs, and parts of the body are cut off from other parts.
- Positions of shoulders and arms. These show the relationship a person has with the world. Hunched shoulders may reflect a protective position. Pulled back shoulders may reflect fear. Figure 5–3B shows hunched shoulders and possibly a protective position.
- Head positions and facial expressions. The head, neck, and face show us the relationship between thinking and feeling. The throat represents the border between the two. Figure 5–3B shows both a forward head position and rounded shoulders. Look for the head forward; it may reflect aggression or determination. Head to the side may reflect indecision or not wanting to meet the world "head on." Jaw line may reflect aggression if jutting out, or if retracted, may reflect a person who is unable to speak out.
- Dominance of the right side—ear or eye larger, right shoulder forward or right foot forward, right pelvis larger and more anterior. Right-sidedness is linked to the left hemisphere of the brain whose task is to be logical, understanding why and how—in general, masculine traits. The right side of the brain and/or the left side of the body represents the creativity, or female traits. Balance is the key here. Figure 5–3C shows a lateral curve of the spine known as scoliosis. It suggests right-side dominance and weaker left-side balance.
- Compression of the rib cage, breathing patterns, and areas of the body where you do not see breathing happening. A plumbline can be used for this purpose (Fig. 5–4). Energy may be blocked where you do not see breathing happening. Feelings are also connected to breathing. An area may be too painful to breathe.

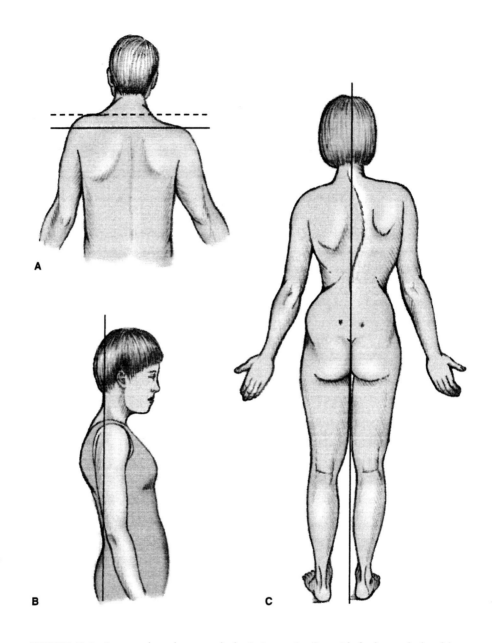

FIGURE 5–3. Structural and postural deviations. **A.** One-sided elevated shoulder. **B.** Forward head and stressed posterior muscles in neck and shoulders. **C.** Scoliosis or lateral spinal curve, showing dominance of right side and weakness in left side.

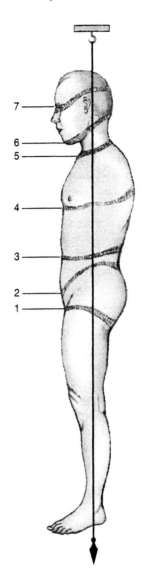

FIGURE 5–4. Plumbline figure with fascial bands. Seven major bands ring the torso while several minor ones can be found around the joints on the extremities.

Current studies at the institute include the effects of massage in the following areas:

- Offsetting the need for addictive pain medications in pediatric pain.
- Depression and adjustment disorder in children and adults. Children were less depressed, stress hormones were descended, and nurses said subjects were more cooperative and nighttime sleep patterns improved.

- Abused and neglected children and children exposed to drugs during pregnancy. Results showed it is as beneficial to touch as to be touched. Volunteer retirees who massaged the children showed a decrease in depression, increased feelings of self-worth, improved sleep patterns, and fewer doctor visits. The children were more responsive following the treatment program.
- Job performance and stress reduction at the University of Miami Medical School. Job stress reduced and productivity increased.
- HIV-positive men to determine the effects on the immune system. After 45 minutes of massage therapy 5 days a week for a month, the men showed decreased anxiety and stress levels and increased levels of natural killer cells, suggesting that they will have fewer opportunistic infections like pneumonia.

One project in process includes a study on a cross-section of humans and their problems. The research efforts clearly show that touch therapy can play an important role in treating diverse medical conditions. "As the medical community continues to investigate alternatives to conventional therapies, ongoing research in touch therapy becomes even more vital" (Field, 1997).

Some interesting studies about touch on hospital patients have revealed physiological changes due to touch. One exciting study, which was controlled for the placebo effect, shows that wounds healed faster in people who received therapeutic touch than in people who did not. Another study showed that blood chemistry can be changed by the laying on of hands or therapeutic touch.

In 1990, the American Massage Therapy Association (AMTA) set up a tax-exempt public charity to promote the development of scientific advances and community services in massage therapy encompassing the areas of research, outreach, and scholarship. Proposals are reviewed once a year in these three categories. Current research, either just completed or under way, includes the programs on the impact of intentional touch on grief, sickle cell pain, alternative approaches to pain control, immunological effects of massage therapy during academic stress, effects of connective tissue massage on migraine, use of massage for cancer pain and anxiety, effects on spasticity of spinal cord injuries, and use of restorative massage to enhance recovery following repetitive swimming events.

The results of the last two studies were available at the time of printing. Clinical implications for the effects of massage on spasticity of spinal cord injuries suggest that petrissage, or kneading, may be used in the clinic to inhibit involuntary motor activity in persons with spinal cord injuries. Spasticity often includes hyperactive tendon jerking and spontaneous spasm, which often interferes with position change, transfers, wheelchair mobility, exercise, and treatment. Petrissage, using one's thumb and forefinger to apply pressure and stretch to the muscle, may be used in the clinic setting to inhibit spasticity selectively.

In the study entitled "Lactate Clearance in Competitive Swimmers: A Comparison of Three Forms of Recovery Following Repetitive, High-Intensity Exercise," active recovery was more effective than either massage or passive recovery. It was noted, however, that athletes would continue to receive massage to help them recover because it made them feel better—and that component might make the difference between winning and losing.

These research projects, and many more, have provided us with the information concerning massage's positive effect on anxiety and stress, its ability to influence the immune system, and its enhancement of adult job performance. Further research has shown that the bonding between caregiver and abused, neglected children is enhanced by massage and that poor sleep habits are improved.

All aspects of human beings need to be kept in balance in research as well as in massage. As research is completed, we can more effectively move massage to a higher professional place among the medical and the alternative therapies being offered to the public.

▪ CASE STUDIES

1. William, a 66-year-old North American Indian, lived on a reserve in Ontario. He came to me in Florida complaining of weak legs, feeling they would not support him. Upon observation, I noticed that the rest of his body looked strong while the legs did not. Using structural alignment methods, we began to work on them so as to balance the torso and the legs. The upper legs did not seem painful to work on and after a treatment or two seemed to be alright. Every time I touched the lower legs, however, William cried out in pain and asked to have the treatment stopped. Even so, the legs responded, and as he saw that, he gave permission to begin again. Eventually, he confided that, as a boy, he had attended an Indian school on the reservation. The English headmaster had been in the military in India and, military style, his punishment for boyish pranks was to hit the lower legs of the boys with willow switches. The deep work of the treatment raised these memories. By using several energetic modalities such as aura stroking and polarity, the legs cleansed themselves and began to feel stronger. We were able to progress through the rest of the treatments without pain.

2. Abuse cases are becoming more frequent in massage as society encourages people to seek help. Although massage therapists are not trained to act as counselors, we can do bodywork and often generally aid the client and work with other professionals for a common goal.

   Helen, age 50 and married with several children, came for bodywork to aid the long search of her abuse memories and to rid the body of early memories. She was already seeing a female psychotherapist who was also a hypnotherapist, and Helen was a member of a support group.

   She had been struggling since early childhood to deal with her abuse, as it had gone on for years and was perpetrated by family members. She had never been comfortable with sexual intimacies with her husband and wanted this to change. Massage helped as different areas of her body responded differently. She and her therapist together arranged to have several joint sessions with the massage therapist. The psychotherapist worked with her during the sessions, using hypnotherapy, while the massage therapist used Swedish massage and sometimes Neuromuscular Integration. All three agreed it was most benficial to work together this way. A lovely footnote to this story is that Helen was so moved by this work that she became a massage therapist and is now working in a private hospital with emotionally disturbed persons.

3. Another interesting case involved a physician's wife, Joan, age 47, who came in to have her neck and shoulders worked on. She had a history of chronic problems across the shoulders and into the neck, along with temporomandibular joint (TMJ) problems. She had been seeing both a physician and a chiropractor but could not seem to clear the problem for good. Early in the first treatment, she began to tell me about building her house for the past few years and the difficulties she had had with the contractor and the builders. It seemed she was in the middle of several lawsuits and giving depositions weekly. It was apparent that this experience had traumatized this area of her body, although no direct injury had caused it.

One of the main functions in the neck is connected to speech. Weakened by previous conditions and subjected to the extreme amount of talking being done, most of it under pressure and stress, that area of her body gave in to the trauma. The whole experience became one big pain in the neck. We worked on several levels at the same time: heat and massage for tired muscles and spasms, finding ways in her life so that she had control of the situation, and positive ways to think about it all. We had minimal success until the lawsuits were ended. Over one week's time, she seemed to make enormous strides towards wellness. Since then, she has come in for TMJ syndrome as it starts to be uncomfortable, but she remains pain free and seems to be more in control of her stress levels.

4. Angela, 35 years old, came in for massage experiencing both kidney and heart dysfunctions. She was under a physician's care but was depressed and spoke about dying. Manual massage was contraindicated while therapeutic touch, done with the hands off the body, was possible with the client sitting in a chair. An assessment of the body's biomagnetic fields revealed hot spots (static energy), warm and cold spots (depleted energy), and uneven areas (energy needing reorganization). Starting from the head and working towards the feet, energy was removed where static, added where depleted, and smoothed out where uneven. Afterwards, the client felt revitalized and began speaking about living. Therapeutic touch works on all levels—physical, emotional, mental, and spiritual.

In all of these cases, something is going on besides just bodily discomfort. Sometimes the mind is noticeably in control, sometimes the body or the emotions. All areas—body, mind, emotions, and spirit—work all of the time and it is hard, of course, to decide which is which. But by treating the whole person and caring deeply about our client's health, massage can do wonders.

REVIEW QUESTIONS

1. Give an example of how the mind might influence the body. How might the body influence the mind?
2. How might the new branch of medicine called psychoneuroimmunology help massage therapists?
3. Why is it so difficult to explain humans in their "wholeness"?
4. Do you think it is good to divide humans into parts for the purpose of studying them? Why or why not? (This does not refer to human dissection.)
5. Discuss the various components of the medical model.
6. Give an everyday example of the body, mind, emotions, and spirit of an individual working together.
7. Give an example of how you think the emotions might or might not be the link between the body and mind.
8. List several modalities that might be classified as energetic approaches.
9. Give an example of the current research referenced in this chapter.
10. Name three things to look for during postural assessment.
11. Tell how the results of the research in Question 9 might help massage.
12. Define the vocabulary terms at the beginning of this chapter.

PREPARATION FOR AND CONSULTATION WITH THE CLIENT

It is much more important to know what sort of a patient has a disease than what sort of disease a patient has.

William Osler

LEARNING OBJECTIVES

After reading this chapter, students will be able to:
1. Describe the atmosphere needed for the best results in massage.
2. Explain how to set boundaries.
3. Formulate questions and dialogue with the client to determine the client's needs.
4. Explain the common elements needed in the client–therapist relationship for successful interaction.
5. Explain the various tissue components assessed by palpation.
6. Explain the components of a treatment plan.
7. Develop a treatment plan for a client.
8. Define the following vocabulary terms.

VOCABULARY TERMS

Consultation   Palpation   SOAP notes

▪ ATMOSPHERE FOR MASSAGE

No matter where massage is given—in a client's home, in an office, or in a clinic-like setting—certain elements are important to the success of the massage treatment (Fig. 6–1). The framework for a successful massage treatment is an atmosphere that creates trust, safety, and confidence. It is the responsibility of the professional therapist to provide that framework by setting and maintaining a clear professional boundary between client and therapist. Both parties must feel safe, respected, and comfortable in the surroundings. The following guidelines for appropriate behavior between therapist and client help to create a safe environment. These were published by Dr. Benjamin in the *Massage Therapy Journal* (1992). (Refer to Appendix B.)

- No sexual contact or intercourse between practitioner and client before, during, or after a treatment session.
- No sexual contact or dating between practitioner and client during the course of treatments.
- If the practitioner and client want to have a romantic relationship, the professional relationship must be terminated first.
- The practitioner is responsible for maintaining appropriate boundaries even if the client is perceived as being seductive.
- Client undresses and dresses in private.
- Client has a clear choice as to whether he or she is nude, wears underwear, or wears a smock during the treatment.
- Practitioner never works on or in the genital area or anus.
- Practitioner never works on the nipple area of a client.
- Practitioner uses only the hands, arms, elbows, and feet to massage a client.
- Practitioner uses only the knee, lateral aspect of the hip, and lower leg for bracing.
- Practitioner never uses the chest, head, face, lips, pelvis, or breasts to massage a client.
- Practitioner does not use inappropriate parts of body for bracing (front of the pelvis, face).
- Appropriate draping procedures will always be observed.
- The practitioner refrains from flirting with clients verbally or otherwise creating a flirtatious atmosphere.
- The practitioner uses appropriate clinical terminology when speaking about body parts to the client.
- The practitioner does not make remarks about client's body that contain sexual innuendo.

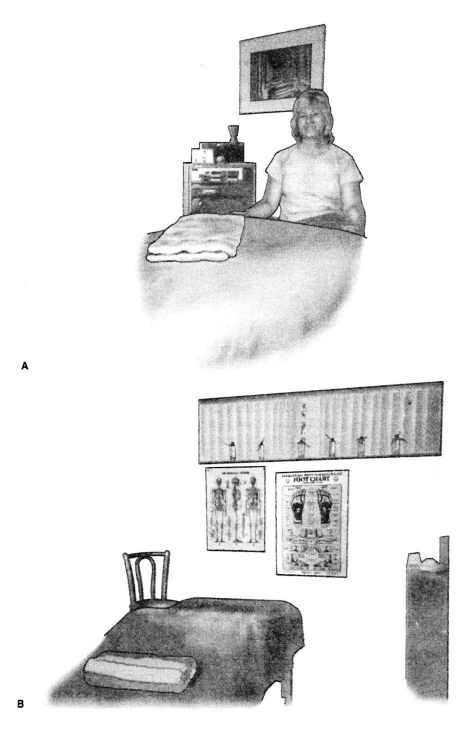

FIGURE 6–1. Room setup in **(A)** a therapist's home and **(B)** in a clinical setting.

- The practitioner does not probe intrusively for information about the client's emotional/sexual history, or in any way imply that the client must give such information.
- If information about the client's emotional/sexual history is communicated, the practitioner does not offer judgments or diagnoses.
- In cases where the practitioner suspects a sexual abuse history that is not perceived by the client, the practitioner refrains from imposing his or her opinion on the client.
- The practitioner must remain within his or her scope of practice and training when dealing with sexual issues. This includes referring to, or working in conjunction with, other practitioners when appropriate for the well-being of the client and bodyworker.
- Practitioner seeks informed consent from the client to work on certain parts of the body. Examples include high on the thigh, on the chest around breast tissue, buttock, front of the hip near the genital area, and the stomach.

Because the therapist is in charge of the treatment session and, usually, the location, with the client being unclothed, the power differential is great. Maximum care is needed to keep social and professional interaction separated. The therapist needs to realize that often clients cannot verbalize or identify their safety zones. Constant feedback is needed during the treatment to help the therapist monitor the situation.

Care must be given to provide a comfortable but professional location for massage. A successful massage can be given almost anywhere. Certainly places of business, airports, factories, corporation offices, sporting events, and health-related and medical massage clinics have all become popular locations. Seated massage is performed in corporate offices, hospitals, nursing homes, factories, and elsewhere (Fig. 6–2). So it appears that along with the clients' hopes, the components that create a professional image are what is important. The more professional the place that you use to give a massage is, the more professional your demeanor will be and the more professional your client will act toward you, the therapist.

▪ DETERMINING THE CLIENT'S NEEDS

Before the massage begins, good communication between client and therapist must take place. This can begin on the phone when the appointment is made. The client needs to explain her or his desires and needs for the massage, and the therapist needs to explain policies and procedures about the massage. Screening the client over the telephone will help eliminate individuals wanting a procedure or outcome that the therapist will not or cannot provide. If this is the case, the client can be referred to another therapist or healthcare provider. Finding out if the client has had massage before, why this treatment session is desired, and who referred the client are easy questions to ask on the phone, and the answers instruct you on how to proceed.

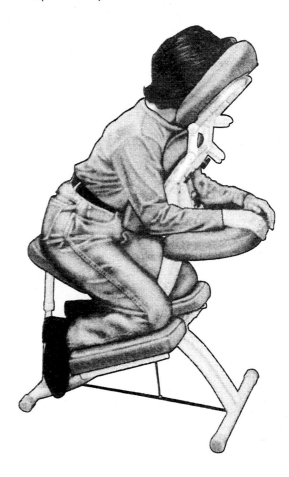

FIGURE 6–2. Seated massage. Body support systems or pillows may be used to create a safe and comfortable massage setting for women after the first trimester of pregnancy.

Before the client arrives, the treatment room should be prepared, linens and draping determined, and records and files made ready. Often the appointment is made with a receptionist or in haste, and then the entire process needs to be done in person during the consultation before the massage.

▪ CLIENT–THERAPIST INTERACTION

Approaching a client for the first time offers a first impression of confidence, competence, and leadership in your role as therapist. An outstretched hand indicates a handshake (and should be a firm grip), or a light touch on the shoulder or arm begins the contact and communication process (Fig. 6–3).

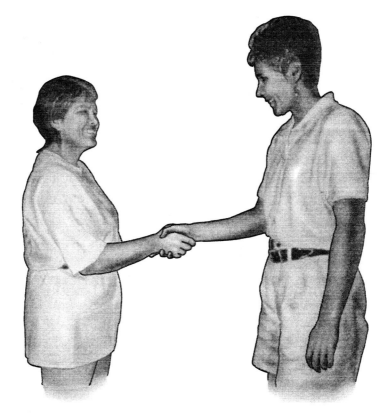

FIGURE 6–3. Approaching the client for the first time. *(Continued)*

Observation of the client begins the fact-finding process that will aid you in deciding on a treatment plan. Posture, vitality, skin tone and texture, eye contact, body type and movement, obvious problem areas, reaction to questions, speech patterns, and attitude are but a few items to observe and note. Introductions and a social greeting begin your verbal communication. Next, you want to give the client a chance to explain his or her desires about massage. Find out if the client has had a massage before. If not, explain your procedures and state the policies that govern your practice. Even if the client has had a massage before, you can explain your procedures and what the client can expect. Never assume that clients know what you do and how it will affect them. A previous cruise ship massage, or one from a friend with no training, are not necessarily the same types of massage, nor will they have the same outcome that a professional therapeutic massage will have.

Items that should be explained in the **consultation,** the meeting between the client and therapist to obtain information concerning the client's health, include the following:

- Services offered and fees.
- Working, if applicable, with insurance companies.

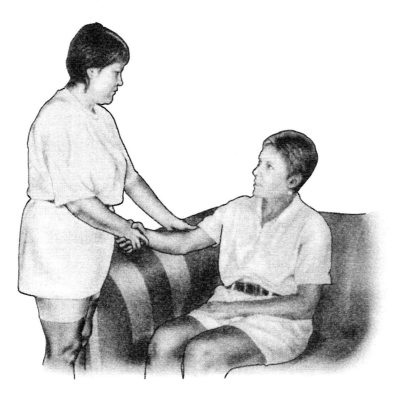

FIGURE 6–3 (cont.).

- Your training and experience and type of massage you perform.
- Appointment, cancellation, and late policies.
- Your work schedule and length of average session.
- Your first visit procedure.
- Dressing and undressing procedures.
- Ask for feedback on your pressure and uncomfortable areas for the client.
- If you offer music, ask for client's preference and discuss lighting levels.
- Once the treatment plan has been formulated and agreed upon, tell the client any changes in the plan will be discussed and consent asked before the change is made.
- Tell the client about your code of ethics (better still, display one) and inform client of confidentiality.
- Discuss the benefits of massage and apply the knowledge to your client's needs.

Once this has been discussed, it is time to take a health history. A client can often fill in the health history form while waiting for you to be available. If that is the case, you can now begin to discuss anything on the form that you need to clarify. You are looking for contraindications, reasons to refer the client to another healthcare practitioner, ways in which massage may help this client, and eventually informed consent from the client about the treatment plan that you design.

Ask questions about previous injuries and surgeries, find out why the client is under a physician's care, and any medications being taken. Ask the client to identify problem areas, points of pain, and the progression of the problem. Ask the clients' profession or job, and about athletic activities or exercise. Ask the client what he or she wants you to work on and discuss options that you think should be considered. Begin to formulate what is realistic to accomplish in the time available, how you should proceed, and what techniques you will use. Get consent for your plan. Further assessment will take place as you palpate the tissue, and a change of plan can be discussed then. Have the client sign a disclaimer, which usually says that you do not diagnose or treat any medical condition. In some areas of the country, treatment-specific plans need to be written for each visit. Be sure to comply with the laws in your area.

▪ PALPATION SKILLS

More information from the client can be obtained by **palpation,** or assessment of the tissue through touch. Sometimes it is logical to feel the tissue in an area while the client is telling you about it. Sometimes it seems better to assess the tissue once the client is on the table, positioned for massage. Whenever it is done, the main function of palpation is to receive information through the therapist's hand from the client's body. Temperature, skin condition, body rhythms, breathing patterns, pulses, and cranial–sacral pulse can be obtained. The levels of skin, fascia, muscles, tendons, ligaments, blood vessels, bone joints, and viscera can be felt and assessed.

When the student is learning palpation skills, it is important to start with superficial tissue and then proceed to the deeper levels, as sensors on the superficial tissue decrease in sensitivity as the touch goes deeper.

▪ DEVELOPING A TREATMENT PLAN

The information gathered from the client's history form, the questioning and discussion of that form with the client, your observations during consultation, and any palpation you have done to this point will allow you to put together a treatment plan. The client's desires and needs should be kept in mind along with your understanding of what can be accomplished in this session. You may also have a long-range plan in mind, but you need a realistic plan for this session. If this is not your first session with this client, your treatment notes from previous sessions (i.e., **SOAP notes**) would certainly be reviewed, too. Options for this session can be discussed with the client, and when you have reached a decision as to what will be done, you need to get informed consent from the client. Consent can be obtained in writing or verbally. In either case, the treatment plan needs to be written in the

SOAP notes. Goals for further sessions may also be included. Which modalities you use in which order needs to be thought through depending upon the desired outcomes. Once you complete your plan and record it, you can begin the massage. Depending on what you find, you can adjust your plan or create a new one. But changing the treatment plan will require you to receive informed consent again from your client.

▪ POSITIONING AND DRAPING THE CLIENT

Positioning and draping a client on the massage table is done for client comfort and for easy access to the body part to be massaged. Various parts of the body can be supported with rolled pillows, folded towels, foam bolsters, or the body support system of various-sized foam wedges and bolsters. Normal areas of the body to be supported are:

- Under the ankles when in prone position (face down).
- Under the knees when supine (face up).
- Under the head as desired.
- Under the abdomen for low back support when prone.
- Under the chest when women are large breasted and lying prone.
- As needed for support and comfort.

Use multiple supports when a pregnant client in the second or third trimester is side-lying (Fig. 6–4). All supports need to be covered with washable material or placed under the bottom sheet for sanitation reasons.

Keeping the client warm, comfortable, and secure are the reasons for draping during a massage. Protecting the boundary between client and therapist is part of maintaining the client's trust. Draping is an important issue in boundary maintenance. General rules for draping include the following:

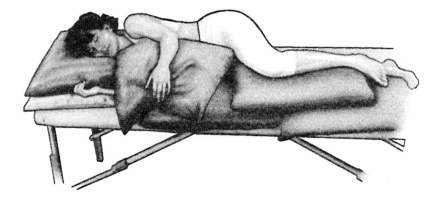

FIGURE 6–4. Side-lying positioning for pregnancy.

1. Only the area to be massaged is undraped (Fig. 6–5).
2. Genital and breast areas are always draped (except when medical or therapeutic breast massage is being performed, and then rule 1 still applies. Special education and training are needed to perform this type of massage. Check local and state laws to see if it is permissible in your area).
3. The client should be covered in all positions. Draping needs to be adequate.
4. All linens need to be clean for each client.

You can use several draping methods:

- A combination of a sheet and a towel for better coverage and easy manipulation (Fig. 6–6A, B).
- Top and bottom sheets as on a bed (Fig. 6–6B).
- Two bath-sized towels: one for a breast towel, one for genital coverage. These can be manipulated for abdominal and pelvic work (Fig. 6–6C).
- Diaper draping (Fig. 6–6C). One towel is gathered between client's legs to cover the genital area, and a second towel is draped across the pelvic region. For a female client, a third towel is used as a breast towel.

Practice is needed to ensure covering and ease of movement when turning a client. Treatment can be done with the client fully clothed. Swimsuits and short shorts may also be worn, but continue to have a covering for warmth.

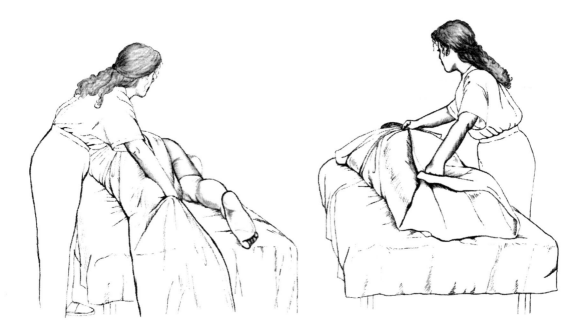

FIGURE 6–5. Draping techniques.

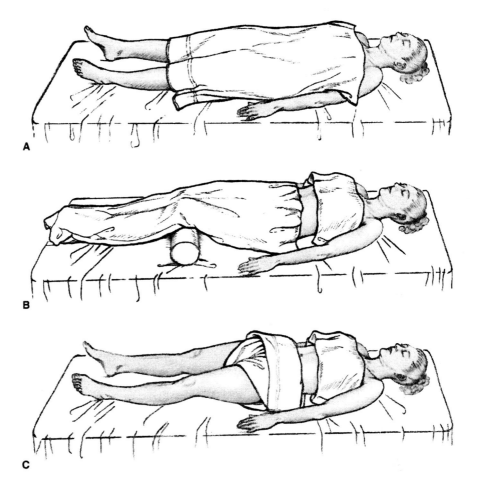

FIGURE 6–6. Types of draping. **A.** Sheet and one towel. **B.** Sheet on the top and bottom plus one towel used as a breast towel. **C.** Diaper draping using two towels.

If a client is undressing in a room away from the massage table, a suitable covering needs to be available for the walk between the two rooms. Terrycloth robes are often used in spas; sarong-type beach coverings are also popular. The latter can be used as the covering while the client has his or her massage. The top covering or robe will also be used by the client to return to the dressing area after the massage.

▪ AFTER THE MASSAGE

If possible, it is beneficial for the client to rest for a short time after the treatment. Help the client off the table and with dressing, if necessary. Arrange the next appointment and collect any outstanding fees. At this time, tell the client anything you want him or her to do before the next appointment. This might be as simple as drinking more water than usual to help flush toxins from tissues, or it might be the use of a hydrotherapy technique or exercises to aid healing. Keep the conversation short and connected to health and healing rather than social. Do not linger; say "goodbye" and make a move to leave them. Return to your treatment room, update your records, and prepare the room for the next client. Now you can relax until your next client arrives.

REVIEW QUESTIONS

1. Discuss the guidelines for safe and ethical contact as presented at the start of the chapter.
2. Describe several elements that create a suitable atmosphere for a successful and professional massage. Discuss what is not suitable.
3. Explain how a therapist can set boundaries between himself or herself and the client.
4. Formulate several questions you might ask a client that will help you determine the client's desires and needs.
5. What are some elements needed for successful therapist–client interaction?
6. Describe the type of forms needed to set up client files.
7. What should be included in a treatment plan?
8. *Class project.* Prepare a list of items to be explained to clients as you usher them into the treatment room for the first time.
9. *Class project.* Prepare a script to be practiced by students in the consultation. Include all the items suggested in this chapter, and add any others you think might be helpful.
10. Practice taking health histories from several people. Then discuss the forms with them and practice formulating a treatment plan.
11. Develop a treatment plan for a client from one of the case studies given in Appendix A.
12. Define the vocabulary terms at the beginning of this chapter.

7

MAJOR MASSAGE STROKES

You don't understand anything until you learn it more than one way.

Marvin Minsky

LEARNING OBJECTIVES

After reading this chapter, students will be able to:
1. Define the seven major massage strokes.
2. Perform the seven major massage strokes.
3. Describe the physiological effects of each of the strokes.
4. Perform stretching exercises.
5. Define the following vocabulary terms.

VOCABULARY TERMS

Compression	Joint movement	Proprioception
Friction	Kneading	Spindle cell
Gliding	Pain threshold	Touch
Golgi tendon organs	Percussion	Vibration

▪ INTRODUCTION

Massage movements or strokes have evolved over time. In ancient Greece, massage strokes were called "rubbing" the skin. By the 1500s, the terms "kneading" and "friction" were added. By the time Per Henrik Ling developed the system of Swedish massage in the 1800s, the strokes were called by their French names and included effleurage, pettrissage, friction, tapotement, vibration, and joint movement. Within the last few years, the French terms have been less commonly used. The more generic or current terms of touch, gliding, kneading, compression, friction, percussion, vibration, and joint movements are now generally used. For the purposes of this book, the current terms will be used.

▪ THE SEVEN BASIC MASSAGE STROKES

Touch is simply placing your hand, forearm, fingers, or palm firmly on the client, with no movement. The therapist is reaching into the personal space of the client and therefore must convey the intent to do no harm. The sense receptors on the client's skin will indicate heat, pressure, air movement, and so forth, and so it is important not to activate the fight-or-flight syndrome. It is also important to indicate to the client that this is safe touch.

Touch may be gentle or deep. Light touch (Figs. 7–1 and 7–8) allows the therapist to show the client safe touch at the beginning of the massage. Deep touch (Fig. 7–9) is usually done after the tissue is warmed, later in the massage.

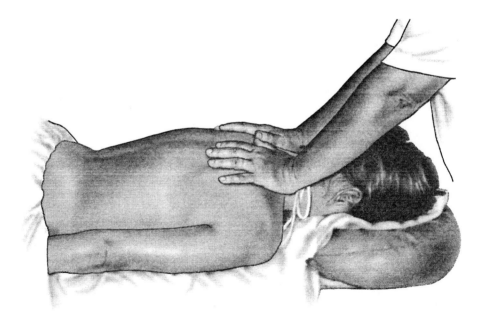

FIGURE 7–1. Light touch is generally used to begin a massage and to acquaint both therapist and client with the other's touch.

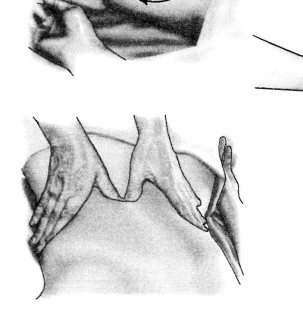

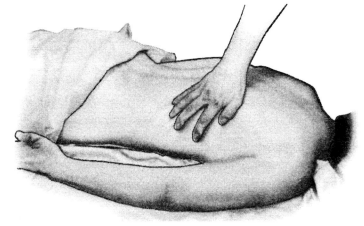

FIGURE 7–2. Gliding strokes are often used to cover large areas of the body, such as the back, to transition from one body part to another, and to stimulate the circulatory or lymphatic systems.

Gliding is the stroking of skin tissue by the hand, fingers, or forearm. Originally, the term "effleurage" meant "to touch lightly." However, the gliding stroke is used both lightly and with increasing pressure, depending on the desired effect. See Figure 7–2 for examples of gliding.

Kneading is vertically lifting, squeezing, and rolling the tissue (Fig. 7–3). The term "pettrissage" means "to knead." **Compression** is part of this stroke, as it is necessary to add pressure or compress the tissue in order to lift it.

Compression is often used in connection with other strokes such as kneading and vibration (Fig. 7–4). However, since sports massage has become popular in

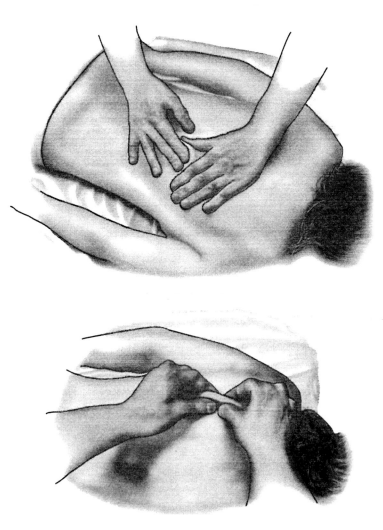

FIGURE 7–3. Kneading strokes are used to lift, knead, squeeze, or roll tissue to detoxify it. *(Continued)*

recent years, it is a stroke that is becoming more popular in its own right. The pressure in this stroke is first downward or vertical into the muscle. Second, there is a lift upwards. Third, there is a downward movement pressing the tissue against the bone. This spreading and squeezing of the tissue softens it. Physiologically, compression stimulates and tones the muscle and stimulates the nervous system. Compression can be done by the finger, thumb, palm, or heel of the hand as well as the fist, knuckle, or elbow.

The therapist using this stroke should take care not to prolong the use of the overextended wrist. Also, the radioulnar side of the elbow should not be used to perform this stroke to avoid pressure on the ulnar nerve.

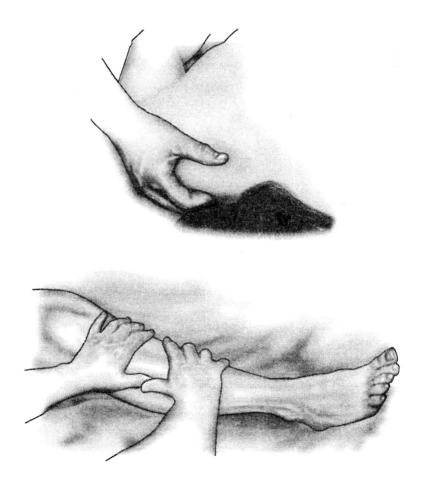

FIGURE 7–3 (cont.). Kneading strokes.

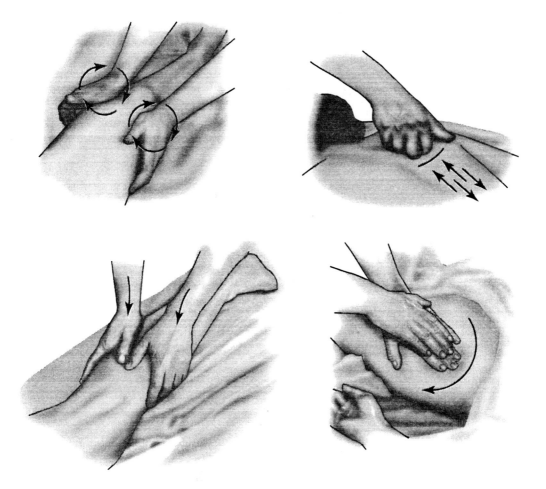

FIGURE 7–4. Compression strokes. *(Continued)*

Friction is the moving of the superficial layers of tissue over the deeper layers. A slight compression or vertical pressing must be done on the top tissue before movement is begun. Movement is generally either cross-fiber or circular. See Figure 7–5 for a variety of friction strokes.

Percussion is striking a series of rapid blows to the body. The blows are directed downward into the tissue using various hand positions, speed, and force. Percussion or tapotement originally meant to drum, pat, or rap. Its purpose is to stimulate. See Figure 7–6 for percussion strokes.

Vibration is a trembling and shaking on a body part used with slight compression or tension on the part before the trembling motion begins. It is difficult to perform successfully and is often used as a nerve stroke. An electrical vibrator is often

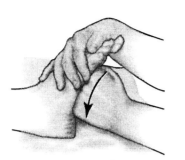

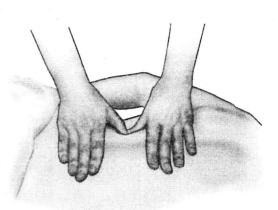

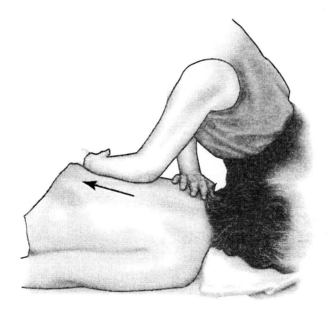

FIGURE 7–4 (cont.). Compression strokes.

used instead of doing the stroke by hand. See Figure 7–7 for examples of vibration strokes.

Joint movement is the systematic movement of a joint through its physiological limits of range-of-motion. It can be done by the client, therapist, or both. Sometimes joint movement is considered with the strokes; sometimes as a separate component. We will assume that knowledge of joint movement is part of your anatomy and physiology training for the purposes of this book.

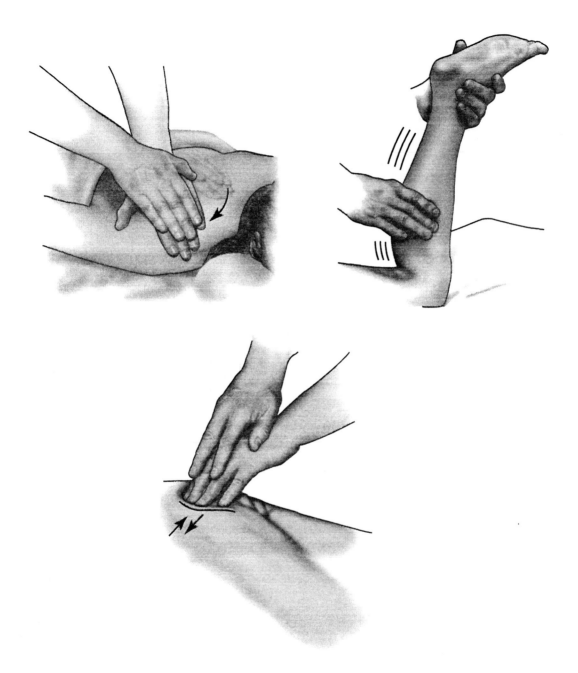

FIGURE 7–5. Friction strokes use the superficial tissue layers to work the deeper layers of tissue. *(Continued)*

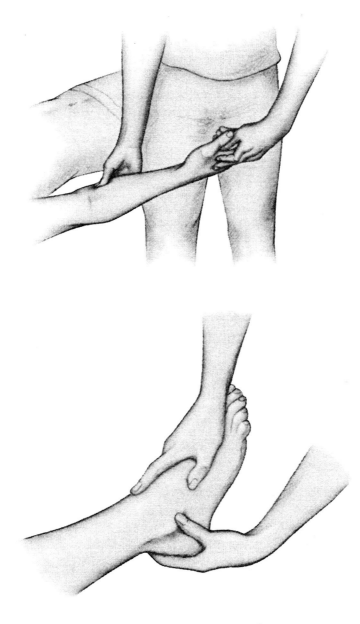

FIGURE 7–5 (cont.). Friction strokes.

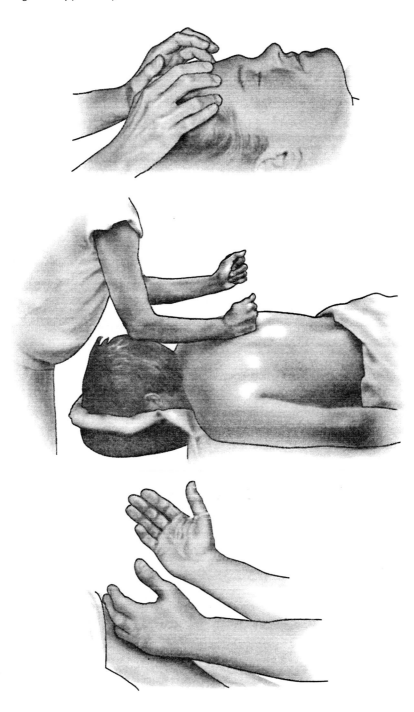

FIGURE 7–6. Percussion strokes are brisk blows to the body in order to stimulate it. *(Continued)*

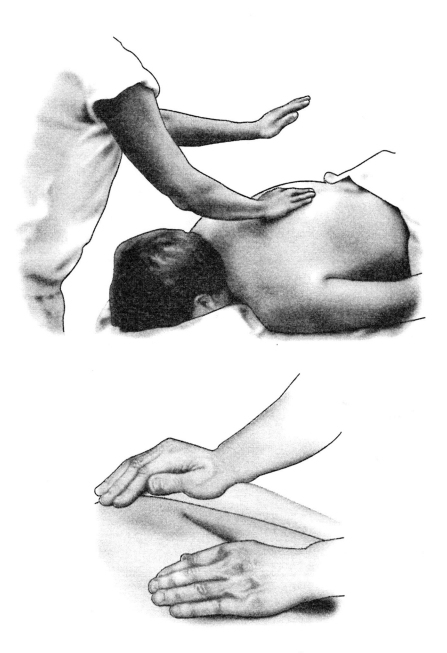

FIGURE 7–6 (cont.). Percussion strokes.

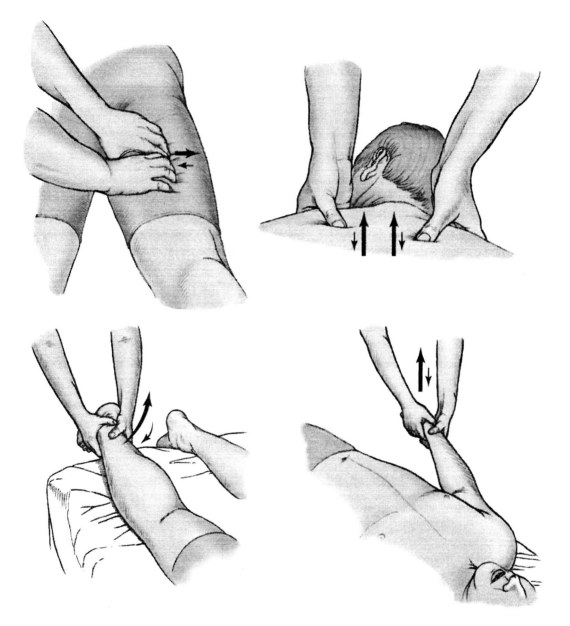

FIGURE 7–7. Vibration strokes are used to shake or tremble a body part and can stimulate or sedate nerves, depending on their use.

▪ APPLICATION OF BASIC MASSAGE STROKES

Touch

The most important tool for communication with a client, touch provides for two-way communication before the other strokes begin and can, indeed, be the first and last contact with the client in the form of a handshake or pat on the shoulder in the waiting room. It conveys to the client the therapist's intent and power. During the massage, touch is continually conveying meaning to and from the client by the therapist and vice versa. Using a resting touch position during the massage allows the client's body a minute or two to catch up with the changes taking place inside the body. Often the heat generated by the therapist's hand held over a problem area is enough to cause change in the tissue. Likewise, asking questions with the hands held over the problem area will often bring intuitive answers from the tissue being worked to the therapist.

The main physiological effect of touch is to soothe. Touch can lower blood pressure, calm the nerves, reassure a client, and begin the healing process. Figure 7–8 shows how a feather stroke may designate the ending of the massage of a particular part.

Deep touch is used when stimulating, anaesthetizing, and calming conditions are needed (Fig. 7–9). Deep pressure is often applied by the thumb, finger, palm of the hand, knuckle, or elbow and is used with other strokes as well. In treatments using reflexology, trigger point, sports massage, or shiatsu, deep pressure is often used. It is important in using any deep pressure that the client is kept below his or her **pain threshold,** the point at which a client feels pain. You can use a client's scale of 1 to 10 to determine where the client is feeling deep touch. The low end of the scale (1) indicates very little or no pain felt, while 10 indicates that you are way over the client's tolerance level. Someplace between 6 and 8 is where "good pain" or mild to medium discomfort exists. Frequent feedback from the client is needed whenever pain is present (Fig. 7–10).

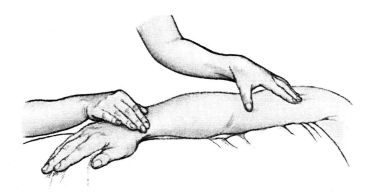

FIGURE 7–8. Light touch. Use of a feather stroke to complete arm massage.

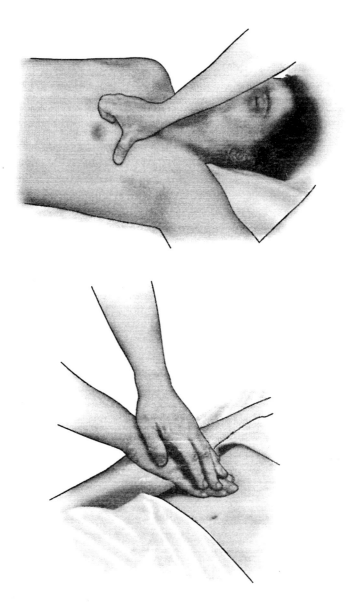

FIGURE 7–9. Deep touch. Deep pressure on a trigger point or a stress point can be accomplished by using thumb, palm, or elbow. Hold the pressure for a short time (30 seconds) and the intensity of the pain will greatly reduce. Be careful that the pressure does not cause the muscle to contract. Never injure the client. *(Continued)*

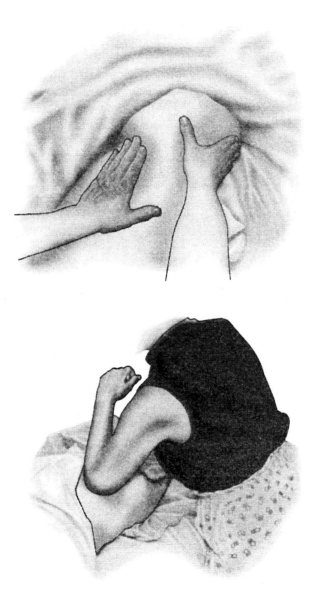

FIGURE 7–9 (cont.). Deep touch.

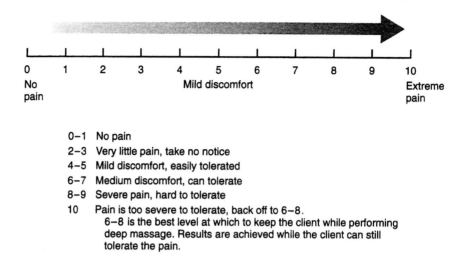

0-1 No pain
2-3 Very little pain, take no notice
4-5 Mild discomfort, easily tolerated
6-7 Medium discomfort, can tolerate
8-9 Severe pain, hard to tolerate
10   Pain is too severe to tolerate, back off to 6-8.
     6-8 is the best level at which to keep the client while performing
     deep massage. Results are achieved while the client can still
     tolerate the pain.

FIGURE 7-10. Client's pain threshold scale.

Gliding

Gliding strokes are used superficially and slowly over the tissue to produce a reflex effect. Gliding strokes are done over the entire body, body part, or area using a variety of pressures. Gliding over the entire body, with the therapist's hand several inches above the body, is called *aura stroking*. Feather stroking (*nerve stroking*) uses very light pressure of the fingertips or the whole hand to create long, flowing strokes. Deeper strokes toward the heart and following fiber direction are mechanical and stimulate blood and lymphatic flow. Moderate to heavy pressure gliding strokes will affect connective tissue and the proprioceptors in the muscle. Heavy pressure produces a compression of soft tissue on the bone. See Figure 7-11 for alternative types of gliding.

Gliding strokes are often used for several reasons:

- As the first and last strokes of massage.
- To spread lubricant.
- To assess the body.
- For continuity between other strokes.
- As a transition stroke from one body part to another.
- To prepare tissue for deeper work.

When using the gliding stroke, the hand should conform to the contours of the tissue being treated and glide smoothly over the body part. The direction is always centripetal, or towards the heart. No pressure is used on the return stroke, although contact is maintained. Remember, slow, rhythmic strokes have a sedative effect, while quick or rapid movements are stimulating.

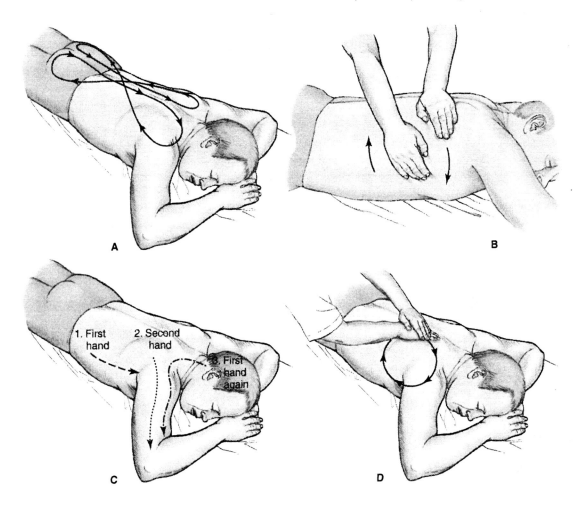

FIGURE 7–11. Alternative gliding strokes include **(A)** the figure 8 stroke, **(B)** horizontal stroking, or shingles, **(C)** the 3-stroke, and **(D)** the hand-over-hand circular stroke.

Kneading

Kneading strokes are used to lift, roll, and squeeze the soft tissue in order to "milk" the fluids and toxins deep inside the muscles. The tissue must be slightly compressed between the thumb and fingers of one hand, or two hands, and then lifted vertically and squeezed as it is rolled out of the hand. The therapist's other hand prepares to lift additional tissue and repeats the movement. Hands are kept flat, contouring to the shape of the body part. This action affects the muscle belly by stretching the spindle cells, and the muscle feels stretched and less stressed. The tendons are stretched, so the whole muscle is "tricked" into feeling relaxed. This stroke also softens and creates space between the fascia layers covering all tissue and can help reduce adhesions. Repeat the movement several times in one spot before moving to another.

Several variations of this stroke exist:

- *Skin rolling* is applied when only the skin and possibly the first layer of fascia needs to be separated from underlying layers of tissue (Fig. 7–12). The fingers and thumb continuously pick up the skin, lift it, and roll the tissue away from the deeper tissue. Areas that appear "stuck" often suggest an underlying problem. This method is often used across the entire back, including across the spine. It is a safe method because it does not affect the deeper tissues investing the spine.
- In *fulling,* the tissue is grasped, lifted, and then spread with the thanar eminence of the thumbs, using the bone as the fulcrum to press the tissue upon (Fig. 7–13).
- In *wringing,* the tissue is grasped, lifted, and then wrung around the bone just as you would wring a washcloth.
- *One-handed kneading* is often used on smaller limbs or on children as well as around the trapezius muscles in the posterior neck. Using the whole hand, the muscle is grasped, lifted away from the bone, and squeezed. You can roll the muscle against itself (Fig. 7–14A).
- The *C or V stroke* is a variation of one-handed kneading. The fingers and thumb form a C or V shape, and the hand is positioned on the distal portion of a limb. The whole hand grasps the tissues and compresses them upon the bone. The pressure is then upwards towards the heart (Fig. 7–14B, C).

Kneading is a very effective stroke for softening, warming, and "milking" the muscle. However, because of its repetitive motion, it is taxing on the therapist and should be used sparingly and only with good body mechanics. By its very nature,

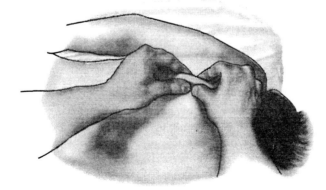

FIGURE 7–12. Skin rolling. Used to lift tissues.

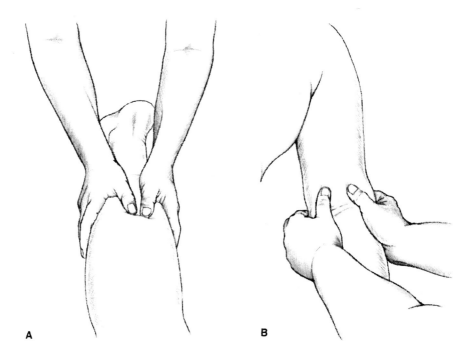

A   **B**

FIGURE 7–13. Fulling. Stroke applied to (**A**) the leg and (**B**) the arm. Tissue is lifted off the bones and then compressed against them.

the speed of a kneading stroke needs to be relatively slow. Often the skin will not roll, making the stroke uncomfortable for the client and hard to perform. Conditions that contribute to making it a difficult stroke include edema, a heavy fatty tissue, adhesions and scarring in underlying tissue, and thickened areas of fascia. Practice is needed to perform kneading in a rhythmic, comfortable fashion for the client. See Figure 7–15 for more variations of kneading.

Friction

Friction is used to reach underlying tissue (Fig. 7–16). Superficial tissue is used to massage deeper tissue by performing small transverse or circular movements with the fingers, thumbs, palms, or elbows. A slight compression of the tissue pressing down vertically facilitates the movement of the deeper tissues. Cyriax's development and use of this method in treatment has made it popular in rehabilitation.

The stroke is usually performed transverse to the fiber direction and can be done for a short time (30 seconds) to a long time (10 minutes). Physiologically, it can break down tissue or produce a slight inflammation response, causing reorganization of the tissue. Friction also causes rehydration of an area in order to keep it soft.

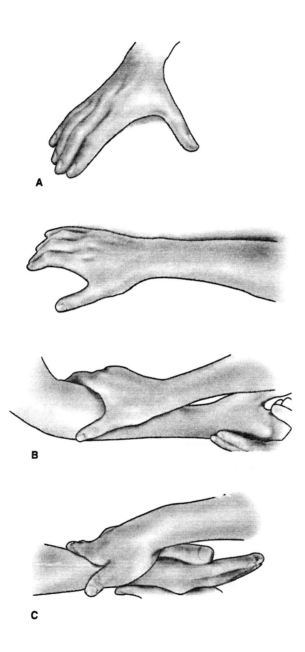

FIGURE 7-14. Alternative kneading strokes include **(A)** the open C-stroke, **(B)** the closed C-stroke, and **(C)** the V-position stroke, used on extremities and neck and shoulders.

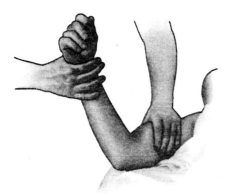

Kneading the upper arm

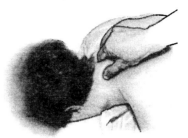

Kneading the posterior neck

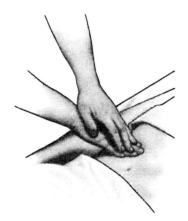

Kneading the abdomen, using
up and down movements

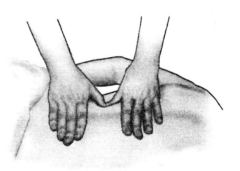

Kneading the back muscles

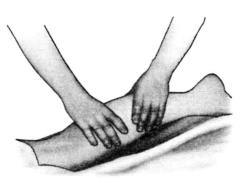

Kneading the lower leg muscles

FIGURE 7–15. Variations of kneading techniques.

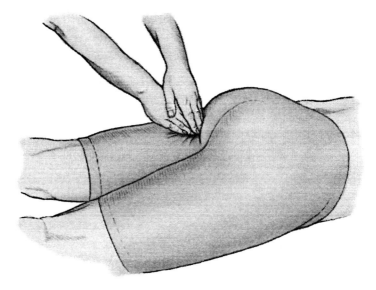

FIGURE 7–16. Cross-fiber friction. Used directly on a lesion site, it encourages soft, pliable scar tissue. On tendons, it reduces rough crystalline deposits that form between tendons and their sheaths.

Friction is often used to access the deep areas in joint spaces and around bony prominences. The areas of musculotendinous junctions are often overused and have connective tissue buildup and adhesions. This stroke is used here to good advantage. Combined with slight compression, friction adds a small stretch to the tissue. It can be used with or without lubricant, but it is done with no sliding.

In *circular friction,* thumb, fingers, and palms compress the tissue slightly and move in a circular fashion. The therapist may press as deeply into the tissues as the client will allow. See Figure 7–17 for several types of circular friction and their uses.

In *cross-fiber friction,* movement occurs across the fiber. This is especially good along the erector spinae or across tendons and ligaments at joints.

As the frictioning movement progresses, it is good to stretch the tissue. This allows the therapist to increase the pressure as the area "lets go." Figure 7–18 demonstrates a fascial stretch. This process may be repeated several times. Another way to facilitate movement is to combine friction with joint movement. Compression to an area is applied, but in place of transverse friction, the body part is moved back and forth or in a circle. Often the therapist as well as the client prefers this type of friction. Its performance seems easier on both therapist and client.

Vibration

Vibration is accomplished by placing a hand on an area of the body, compressing it to the depth desired, and trembling the hand back and forth, transferring the vibration to the tissues. The therapist's forearm is tense, with only the muscles above the

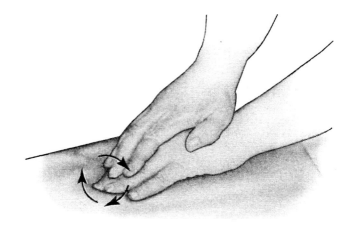

FIGURE 7–17. Circular friction applied along both sides of the spine.

elbow moving. The repetitive quick movements back and forth produce the vibration. Unfortunately, this is a difficult and tiring stroke to do properly. See Figure 7–19 for ways of varying this stroke. To avoid repetitive motion problems, this stroke should be done sparingly. In some instances, a mechanical vibrator will perform the stroke just as well or faster than a therapist can. Three types of vibrators are popular with therapists: orbital (circular), oscillating (side-to-side), and percussion–compression, which produces a "thumping" action (Fig. 7–20).

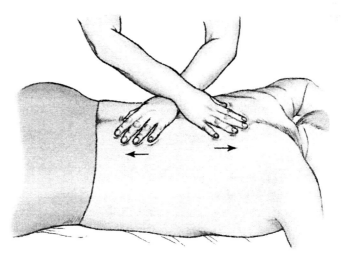

FIGURE 7–18. Fascial stretch using light compressive force.

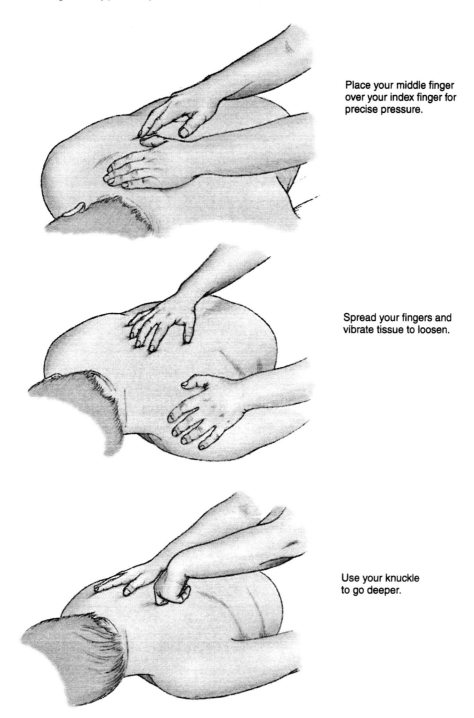

Place your middle finger over your index finger for precise pressure.

Spread your fingers and vibrate tissue to loosen.

Use your knuckle to go deeper.

FIGURE 7–19. Variations of vibration strokes.

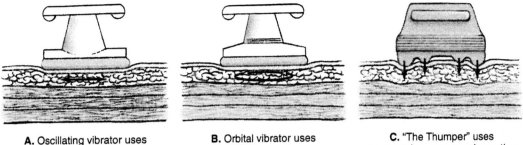

A. Oscillating vibrator uses
a back and forth action

B. Orbital vibrator uses
a circular motion

C. "The Thumper" uses
a percussion–compression action

FIGURE 7–20. Three types of vibrators are sometimes used to aid the therapist in loosening stuck tissue.

When vibration movement is done correctly, it produces a relaxing, sooth-ing effect on the nerves. However, when used with pressure, it is stimulating. When not done correctly, or continued for a prolonged time, it can numb the nerves.

Shaking is a variation of vibration that is useful for clients who have difficulty relaxing. Pick up a limb or large muscle mass, grasp, lift (take the slack out of it), and shake it gently. Focus on the joint and move it within its limit of range-of-motion and the give of the tissue (Fig. 7–21).

Rocking is similar to shaking but is a side-to-side movement without the quick movement at the end of the shake. Rocking the body to and fro is a great assessment tool. The movement should flow, but it shows you where it is sluggish to move. You can rock the body away from you or pull it towards you. See Figure 7–22 for rocking techniques. With a tense, aggravated client, use more gross movements; as the client relaxes, switch to finer rocking movements.

Percussion

Percussion means to strike or tap the body, but the stroke should be performed with-out much force. Quick blows performed by alternating hands striking the body stim-ulate the nerves. Performed on tendons, they stretch. Mechanically, the blows can loosen and move mucous in the chest. They contract superficial vessels on the skin and dilate vessels when performed heavily. Performed on joints, the muscles tense and are stimulated. When used over motor points, percussion stimulates the nerves to fire.

To perform percussion, the open hands are held parallel to each other with wrists relaxed. Alternatively, the third, fourth, and fifth fingertips of each hand strike the body and return to the air in a rapid fashion. Variations include the fol-lowing (Fig. 7–23).

- *Hacking* is done on larger areas such as the back, shoulders, and upper legs with both hands held open. Only the ulnar side of the hand or the little finger hits the tissue.

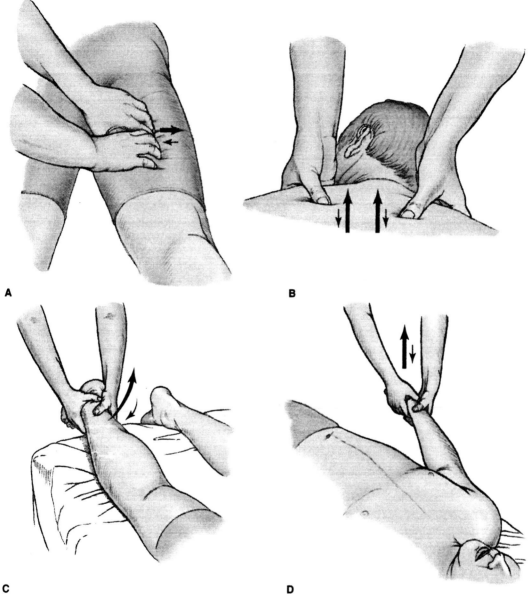

FIGURE 7–21. Shaking techniques. **A, B.** Lift tissue and shake. Return. **C, D.** Pull out slack in tissue and then shake. Return tissue.

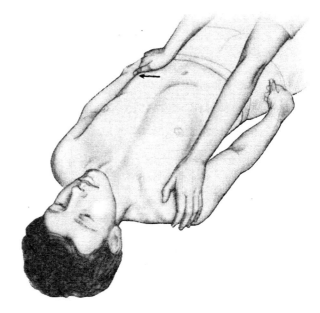

FIGURE 7–22. Rocking technique. Pull area toward therapist, and then push area away from therapist to rock.

- *Slapping* is done with the flat palm of the hand with the fingers or palm making contact with the tissue.
- *Beating* is done with the hand made into a soft fist and hitting the tissue on the ulnar side of the palm. This is usually done on the buttocks and heavy leg muscles.
- *Cupping* is helpful in respiratory illnesses with a buildup of mucus. The cupping is done to aid the client in expectoration. Cupping is done with the hands forming a cup (as in swimming) and using the palmar cup to strike the tissue. This stroke is done on the anterior and posterior thorax to loosen and move congested mucus. Listen for a hollow, loud sound. Often the client will begin to cough while this stroke is performed. Allow the client to expectorate the mucous and repeat the action again. Positioning for cupping is shown in Figure 7–24.
- *Tapping* is done with the palmar surface of the fingers for light to medium pressure. This is a light method used often on face and scalp and along the spine (Fig. 7–25).

Heavy percussion should never be used over the kidneys or in an area experiencing pain. Caution should be used over the heart area.

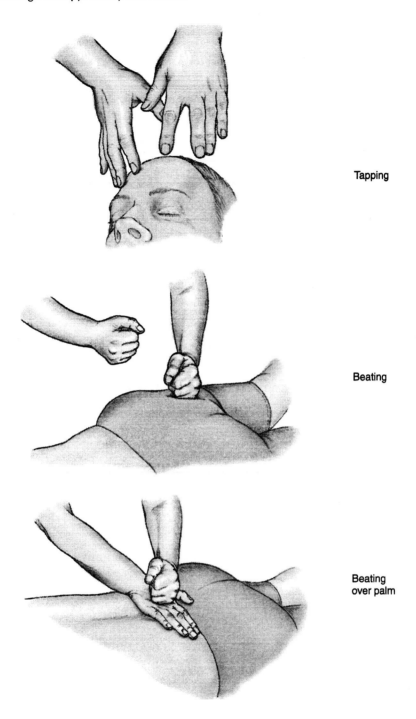

Tapping

Beating

Beating
over palm

FIGURE 7–23. Percussion strokes. *(Continued)*

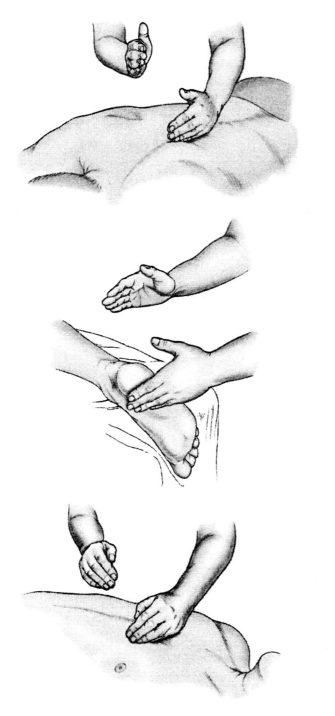

Hacking–
the ulnar side of the
hands follows muscle
fiber direction

Slapping–
a type of tapotement

Cupping–
a type of tapotement

FIGURE 7–23 (cont.). Percussion strokes.

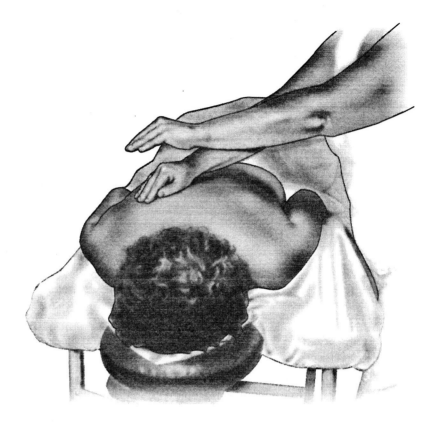

FIGURE 7–24. Positioning for cupping stroke.

▪ PROPRIOCEPTION IN BODY TISSUE

Receptors throughout the body sense the body's movement, location, and relationship to the environment. This information helps the brain to know how the body is functioning. The receptors are usually classified into three types.

- *Exteroceptors* sense touch, cutaneous pain, heat, cold, smell, vision, and hearing.
- *Interoceptors* respond to changes in the viscera, such as pain, hunger, or thirst.
- *Proprioceptors* carry sensations of position, balance, and muscle sense. (**Proprioception** refers to the body's awareness of position, posture, movement, and changes in equilibrium.)

Proprioceptors respond to an inner sense of position and movement, including the positions of muscles and the contractions being made by the muscles. Proprioceptors are located in fasciae, muscles, joints, and tendons. Muscle **spindle cells** and

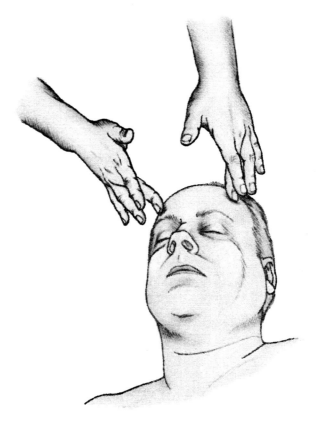

FIGURE 7–25. Tapping stroke used on the head.

Golgi tendon organs are two types of proprioceptors that send messages to the brain stem (Fig. 7–26).

Spindle cells, located in the belly of muscles, detect, evaluate, report, and adjust the length of the muscles in which they lie. The spindles lie parallel to the muscle fibers and can be either described as a muscle bag fiber or a chain fiber. A receptor in the center, called an annulospiral receptor (or primary ending), discharges rapidly and responds quickly to minute changes in muscle length. The secondary ending fires only when larger changes in muscle length occur. The information sent from the muscle includes muscle length, degree of stretch, and speed of movement.

The Golgi tendon receptors and the Golgi tendon end organs, located at musculotendinous junctions, send information of tension and joint activity to the brain independently of the muscular contraction. If excessive overload on the joint is detected, the muscle may cease to function to prevent damage.

Thus, every body part is monitored and information sent to the brain, where it can be integrated for total body awareness. Due to the complexity of the reporting

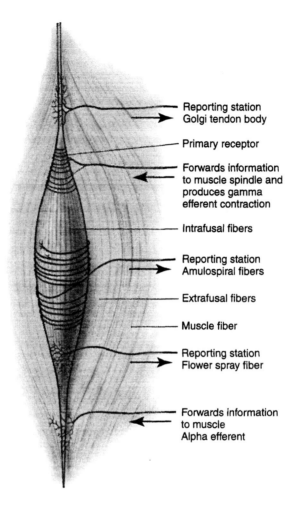

Reporting station
Golgi tendon body

Primary receptor

Forwards information
to muscle spindle and
produces gamma
efferent contraction

Intrafusal fibers

Reporting station
Amulospiral fibers

Extrafusal fibers

Muscle fiber

Reporting station
Flower spray fiber

Forwards information
to muscle
Alpha efferent

FIGURE 7–26. Muscle spindle cell showing Golgi tendon organ and neural pathways.

system, however, conflicting information may be recorded in the brain, at which time no adequate response would occur. Most likely, activity would stop and the muscle might spasm or splinting might occur.

The transmission through the central nervous system of perceived pain is a complex process. The dorsal horn of the spinal cord acts like a computer that processes the incoming sensory signals, rearranging and modulating them before sending them to a higher level. The signal of pain from the muscle or skin to the brain cortex is transformed at least four times and on at least four levels. It can modulate the signal at the receptor that converts the stimulus into nerve impulses, at the spinal cord level, in the relay stations between the spinal cord and the sensory cortex (thalamus), and in the sensory cortex itself.

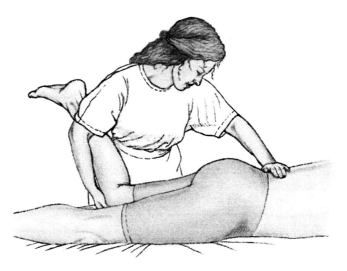

FIGURE 7–27. Strain–counterstrain technique. The therapist uses the legs of the client to find a less painful position to treat an extension strain of the lumbar spine.

Several massage techniques can modify the perception of pain. Neuromuscular techniques work directly with the shortened muscle length. Applied directly on the belly of the muscle, they interrupt and change pain transmission; the muscle relaxes, stops contracting, and lengthens. Muscle energy techniques (MET) produce modifications in the Golgi tendon organ in muscles. Positional release (PR) techniques such as strain–counterstrain (SCS) change soft tissue by modifying the responses of the spindle cells (Chaitow, 1996). Figure 7–27 shows the strain–counterstrain technique.

▪ STRETCHING AND LENGTHENING

Stretching is a mechanical exercise that elongates the muscle to increase or maintain the full use of range-of-motion movements. This protects the muscle from overstretching. Before stretching, lengthening of the muscles must be done or the protective reflex of the spindle cells in the belly of the muscle and close to the muscle/tendonous junction Golgi tendons will counteract the stretching and cause the muscle to spasm.

Longitudinal stretching moves the body in the direction of the fibers and works with a joint. Cross-directional stretching moves the tissue against the direction of the fibers and does not depend on joint movement. The stretching of fascia warms it and makes it soft. Figure 7–28 shows longitudinal stretching of the quadriceps.

Cross-directional stretching in a diagonal direction pulls the muscle fibers against the fiber direction and does not need joint movement to accomplish stretching. Methods used may be strain–counterstrain or positional release, proprioceptive

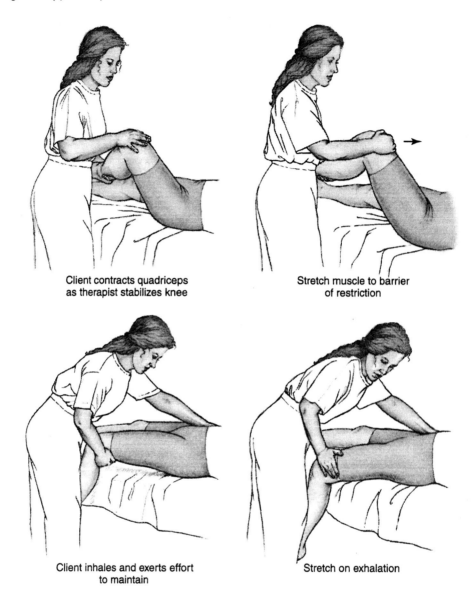

Client contracts quadriceps
as therapist stabilizes knee

Stretch muscle to barrier
of restriction

Client inhales and exerts effort
to maintain

Stretch on exhalation

FIGURE 7–28. Longitudinal stretching.

neuromuscular facilitation (PNF), or muscle energy techniques. Ballistic stretching is not suggested except for the trained athlete, because it depends on explosive, rapid, bouncing movements. Moving against the elastic limits of a joint in this way may result in injuries. Sustained, steady, slow movements against the restrictions of the joint produce the best, safe stretching. The safe rule to follow is to always work under the client's pain threshold.

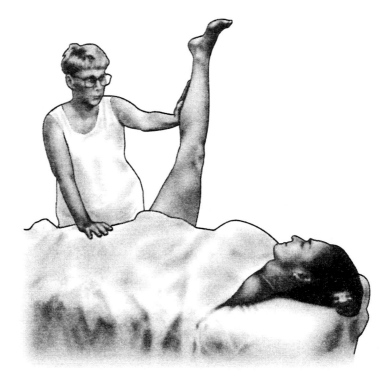

FIGURE 7–29. Stretching techniques can be used after muscles and tissues are loosened or as a method to reset the spindle cell reflex.

General directions for stretching are as follows:

1. Isolate muscles and fibers to be stretched.
2. Choose a method to prepare the muscle to be stretched. See Chapters 8 and 10 for more information.
3. Release soft tissue.
4. Stretch muscle to its limit. (For cross-directional stretching, add twist and pull into restriction.)
5. Hold at its barrier for 10 seconds, take up slack, and repeat to reset the stretch reflex. Hold for 20 to 30 seconds. See Figure 7–29 for another stretching technique.

▪ CONTEMPORARY THERAPEUTIC MASSAGE APPROACHES

This section summarizes the strokes listed in Chapter 8 under each of the modalities referenced there. To understand each stroke thoroughly, read Chapter 8 first and then attempt to discuss and practice each of the strokes. Reread Chapter 8 when you reach it again for a better understanding of the totality of massage and the great diversity of options you have in treating clients and in matching their needs to your skills. When discussing the case studies in Appendix A, use these strokes when appropriate to increase the effectiveness of your skills using both Swedish massage and a variety of other skills needed by your clients. Be creative in meeting the needs of your client.

These strokes and techniques are listed in alphabetical order.

Acupressure or Trigger Points

Acupressure or trigger point work uses a direct pressure with finger or thumb on a sensitive point in the muscle and then a stretch to release the tissue. Pressing the belly of the muscle together may also release the trigger point. It is generally thought that after the trigger point is released, circulation improvement techniques should be used on the area. Acupressure techniques are applied along the meridian lines of the body, near the origin and insertions of the muscles.

Aromatherapy

Using essential oils has advanced over the past several years from a way to release stress and tension to an art form for emotional well-being. Choose the relevant oil for your client, add it to your massage oil, or use it in a diffuser during treatment. Learn as much as you can about the properties of the various oils before blending and using them. Match them to the needs of your clients (Fig. 7–30).

As a general essential oil dosage, use the following:

- *Baths:* 8 drops (do not use basil, cinnamon, clove, peppermint, thyme).
- *Diffuser in air:* 1 to 6 drops in water.
- *Massage oil:* 1 drop to each mL of base oil.
- *Pillows:* 1 to 3 drops.
- *Light bulb ring:* 4 to 6 drops.
- *Lotions and creams:* 10 to 15 drops per 50 mL (1.7 oz).

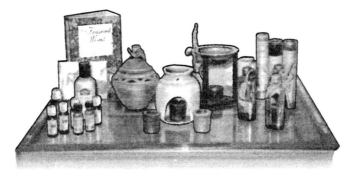

FIGURE 7–30. Aromatherapy accoutrements used by a massage therapist.

Breathing and Relaxation Techniques

Encourage your client to breathe deeply using the abdomen and diaphragm to increase oxygen intake and the circulation of oxygen to all body parts. This increased oxygen will reduce anxiety and stress, decrease the perception of pain, and promote relaxation. If an area of the body is under duress and the therapist is having difficulty loosening the soft tissue, having the client bring his or her breath to the area being worked will aid in clearing the tissue. This is especially important when an emotional component is present.

Connective Tissue Techniques

Move the tissue multidirectionally either into restriction and wait for a change (direct technique), or into the area where the tissue wants to go (indirect technique). Skin rolling, deep stroking, stroking along a restriction, trigger point work, and accupressure are all used. The thumb is used to assess and treat an area as well as the bear claw hold (fingers touching the tissue, palm arched in the air). A stroke or glide of short length (2 to 3 inches) may be repeated several times, going deeper as repeated. Cross-fiber friction to muscle–tendon junctions will aid most trigger points. A T-bar may be used to palpate areas. Stretching and lengthening a body part or tissue creates space and loosens the area. Cross-handed stretching after loosening an area lengthens the tissue in several directions.

Cranial–Sacral Technique

Light pressure (5 grams) is used to cup or hold the body part. The cranial–sacral rhythm is felt while holding the body part, and change is created by stopping the flow of the cranial–sacral system and making the correction needed by using tissue drag. This system allows the therapist to interface with the client's central nervous system. While ordinarily engaging the skull, the spinal cord and fluid within, this method may also be used to determine membrane tension and motility in areas such as the thoracic outlet, diaphram, soles of the feet, and neck.

Hydrotherapy Techniques

Baths, sprays, compresses, and contrast methods can soften tissue before massage, reduce pain, and improve healing. Chill-and-stretch or spray-and-stretch vapocoolants (not environmentally friendly) may be used as well to help deactivate a trigger point. The objectives are to keep the surface of the skin dry, and to chill the surface tissues containing the trigger points but not the muscle. Stretch the underlying muscle. Ice can be used to chill the tissue, but a frozen soft drink can works as well. If you are using a vapocoolant, spray from at least 2 feet away so that the jet stream hits the body at an acute angle. This will lessen the shock. Apply in one direction only and repeat once or twice. See Figure 7–31 for the stretch position and palpation technique. Gently stretch the muscle with the trigger point. The client moves into the restricted area. Repeat several times. The goal is to remove all the trigger points and to regain normal range-of-motion (Fig. 7–32).

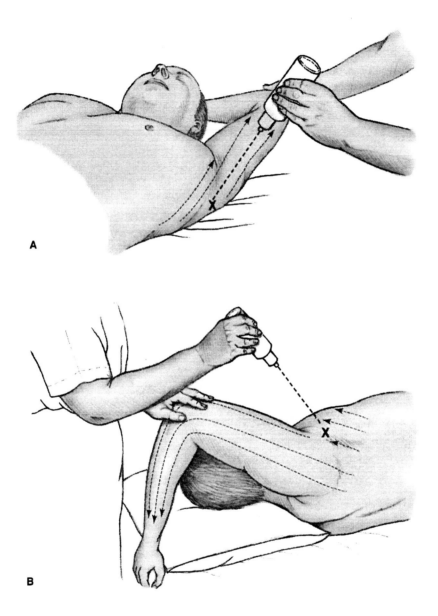

FIGURE 7–31. Chill and stretch and spray and stretch. The stretch position for a trigger point X in the teres major muscle. **A.** Anterior position. **B.** Side position.

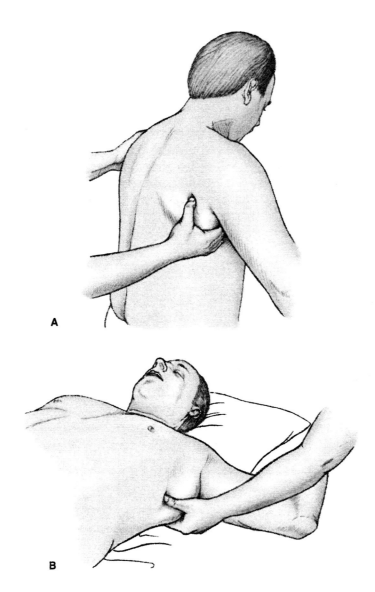

FIGURE 7–32. The therapist must fully encompass the latissimus dorsi muscle to reach the teres major. **A.** Client seated. **B.** Client supine.

Joint Play Technique

The joint play technique is quite different from passive rhythmic movements. Here the emphasis is on the minute movements within the joint, not the whole joint. A passive stretch is given to the small movements in the joint when a restriction is found. Slow, even stretches are applied rhythmically to allow the joint to respond. Joint proprioceptors will then reprogram the muscles crossing the joint, and tone will be reduced. This technique may be used to assess the joint as well.

Manual Lymph Drainage Strokes

Use light pressure on the limb area and overlap small gliding strokes or spiral strokes from proximal to distal areas. Compression strokes to lymph nodes first on the proximal limb with edema will activate and help filter. In larger areas, use stationary circles between an edemic site and proximal nodes. Reduce proximal edema before working distal tissue to ensure good mechanical effects.

Muscle Testing

Muscle testing (touch for health) or applied kinesiology may be used to assess muscles for their strength and function. Then massage techniques, strengthening exercises, or treating by holding accupressure points can assist that muscle to remove energy blockage and clear the tissue. A routine for testing the muscles follows:

1. Isolate the muscle you want to test.
2. Place the extremity or body part in a position so that the ends of the muscle are closer together.
3. Press the body part in a direction that requires the muscle being tested to work to hold the body in position.
4. As you pull the muscle, the client resists the movement. If the muscle is strong, it will lock and stay in place. If the muscle is shaky or feels mushy or gives way, it is weak and needs to be balanced.

Myofascial Release Stroke

Both direct and indirect spreading techniques are used. Deep, long gliding strokes, sometimes called "ironing," are performed using palms, fists, and forearms, and engaging various layers of fascia, spreading and lengthening it. Lifting the tissue is done more often than compression. A twisting motion may also be used. Sometimes the elbow is used working close to the spine but not pressing on the spinous processes.

Neuromuscular Techniques

Neuromuscular techniques reduce pain, fatigue, depression, and stress; they increase mobility. Some of the strokes are the following:

- *Gliding.* Usually with the thumb, light pressure is used to assess the fascia; and deeper pressure is used later to stretch the fascia and release adhesions.

- *Compression.* Pressure is held on painful spots and trigger points, generally 8 to 12 seconds. Always work below the client's pain threshold. Remember, we do not want to cause additional trauma or injury.
- *Skin rolling.* The skin is picked up and rolled to separate the various layers.
- *Stretching.* Stretching is done after tissue is loosened. The muscle and connective tissue involved need to achieve their normal resting length. This is accomplished with active and passive stretching. MET may also be used.

Regular exercise may also be used as client self-care if needed.

Oriental Therapies

Eastern techniques often use accupuncture points along meridian lines to free blocked energies or to balance the body. Follow the directions in which the meridians flow. Six basic strokes are used:

- Light pressure to stroke or rub.
- Rubbing and kneading.
- Small rotations by the thumb.
- Pinching, squeezing, and kneading.
- Vibration.
- Tapping.

Passive Rhythmic Movements (Trager®)

Rocking and shaking movements to a joint are done to loosen the joint in order to normalize it, or to assess the joint. Slight tractioning or stretching the whole joint precedes the shaking or rocking.

Reflexology

Reflexology may be used on hands, feet, or ears to work on areas of the body and the organs. The stroke is performed with the thumb, using an inchworm movement across various points in the foot. See Figure 7–33 for hand position.

RICE

Rest, ice, compression, and elevation (RICE) is used in soft tissue injuries, strains, and sprains. Rest allows the body to begin to regenerate after trauma. Ice (cryotherapy) lessens secondary injury and edema caused by primary injury and keeps the primary injury from getting worse by decreasing metabolism. Compression increases outside pressure, thus controlling edema, and promotes the reabsorption of fluids. Elevation reduces circulation and fluid flow to the injured area. (See also "Hydrotherapy Techniques" earlier in the chapter.) Ice can be applied as follows:

- Ice massage with iced popsicles or frozen cups of ice.
- Ice packs or bags, such as ziplock bags of ice, or frozen vegetable bags.
- Immersion in iced water.

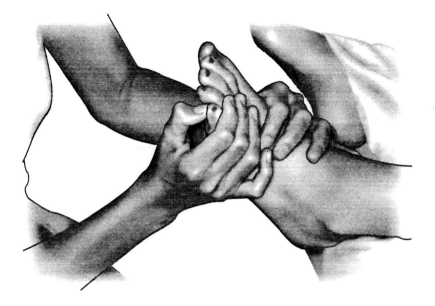

FIGURE 7–33. Reflexology hand position.

- Chemical cold packs.
- Cold whirlpool.
- Cold gel packs (use with caution).

Seated Massage

Many Swedish techniques as well as other modalities can be used in a seated massage, provided over clothing. Many techniques have also been adapted from athletic massage. The following is a list of some of the adapted strokes:

- Friction—use thumb, knuckles, palm around bony prominences.
- Compression—use with twisted movement into tissue.
- Short gliding strokes with slight compression to assist movement over clothes.
- Pumping movement on joints—use palm.
- Wringing or kneading, fulling.
- Rocking, shaking, vibration.
- Bear claw grasp with fingers, twist and move tissue (King, 1993).

Strain–Counterstrain Techniques

Several methods position the body part to be treated in a comfortable position and use the patient's own muscular efforts to create contraction in the specified muscle. Positional Release, MET, and INIT are known as gentle techniques. The therapist applies a counterforce to meet and overcome the patient's force. The muscle is stretched just to the point of irritation, then shortened to reduce the pain. Compression is added and held for 90 seconds. The client is returned to a neutral position and reassessed.

Stroking or Energy Brushing

Stroking or energy brushing techniques are used just off the body, 1 to 4 inches away, to affect the energy system. The pattern for stroking follows the energy flow down the right anterior side of the body and up the back. On the left, it is reversed. Down the right arm and up to the head, up the left arm and to the head. Long gliding strokes are used above the body both to assess the energy flow and to correct the interruption of the energy, if needed. Using the hands to direct the flow, the therapist can direct the energy from one part of the body to another, or to smooth out the energy if it is erratic. Thin spots or depressions in the energy can be filled in with short quick strokes that direct the energy where needed.

Structural Positioning

When therapy includes a structural alignment component, positioning the client in the correct alignment position during the work will help reeducate the body and aid its return to a realigned state. After tissue is released, loosened, and softened with various myofascial and other techniques, the therapist can mold the body and fascial sheaths into the position you and it want to go.

Please read Chapter 8 for more complete information on each of these techniques and systems.

■ CASE STUDIES

1. Anne, in her 40s, liked to entertain her husband's business partners at wine and cheese parties. Often, afterwards, she had moderate migraine headaches and came for massage.

    Suggest a Swedish massage plan for her, including the number of visits and the length of massage. Suggest non-Swedish techniques that can be used in connection with the Swedish massage.

2. Ben, a retired pilot in his late 60s, sustained many injuries during his career due to plane crashes. Now he has aches and pains that, depending on his activities, may travel around the body. He comes regularly for massage.

    Suggest a treatment plan for Ben, addressing areas of soreness and pain. Suggest non-Swedish techniques that can be used in connection with Swedish massage.

3. Ted, age 32, is an amateur athlete who works out in the gym regularly, is in good physical condition, and occasionally runs in local races. He has never had a massage but is interested in the Oriental approach to life. He inquires about the types of massage offered and the benefits of each type. His only problem is a weak ankle, which is not hurting now but sometimes does hurt.

Plan a Swedish massage treatment for Ted, including an assessment of the ankle and treatment of it. Plan an Oriental treatment for Ted, including an assessment of the ankle and treatment of it. (You may need to refer to Chapter 3 and/or the Oriental section in Chapter 8.)

REVIEW QUESTIONS

1. Define the seven basic massage strokes and tell how they are performed.
2. Describe the physiological effects of each of these strokes.
3. Perform all seven basic massage strokes correctly in the presence of an instructor.
4. How do massage techniques affect proprioception in body tissue?
5. Discuss the difference between stretching and lengthening exercises.
6. Use several of the stretching and lengthening techniques in the presence of an instructor.
7. Describe several specialized non-Swedish strokes that can be used in conjunction with Swedish massage.
8. Use several of the specialized non-Swedish strokes in a massage in the presence of an instructor. Ask for evaluation.
9. Define the vocabulary terms at the beginning of this chapter.

CONTEMPORARY THERAPEUTIC MASSAGE APPROACHES

To cure sometimes, to relieve often, to comfort always.

Anonymous

LEARNING OBJECTIVES

After reading this chapter, students will be able to:

1. Describe and discuss the following therapeutic approaches now current in the United States and Canada:

Acupuncture and acupressure	Myofascial techniques
Oriental techniques	Neuromuscular techniques
Connective tissue or fascial techniques	Orthobionomy
Cranial–sacral techniques	Reflexology
Do-in	Seated massage
Fascial Kinetics	Structural alignment
Integrated touch	Trager® technique
Manual lymphatic drainage	Trigger point
Muscle energy techniques	Vibrational energy therapies

2. Demonstrate the use of various strokes from the modalities listed.
3. Determine which specialties suit which style of massage in order to fit the therapist's techniques to the client's needs.
4. Define the following vocabulary terms.

VOCABULARY TERMS

Acupressure	Meridian	Reciprocal inhibition
Acupuncture	Meridian line	Tsubos
Chi (qi, ki)	Moxibustion	Yin and yang
Ground substance	Piezoelectric current	

▪ INTRODUCTION

Specialties in massage have proliferated in the past few years. Every time you read the various magazines of the profession, you encounter something new. It is interesting that the evolution of massage in our time is keeping pace with its growth in popularity . . . or is it the other way around? In any case, there certainly is a modality or two for everyone's presentation.

The following discussion in no way seeks to cover the field. The mere size of a book defines the limit for the author. However, the discussion covers a wide range: soft and hard modalities, those easy to learn and those more challenging, those that can be mastered quickly and those that take longer. The specialties sometimes overlap and can be placed in one or more of the categories listed. Where this is the case, the reader should become familiar with both of the categories that apply.

Michael Shea once said at a graduation of massage students that massage therapists would do well to learn three modalities well, master each in turn, and apply them successfully in their practices. He likened such mastery to filling a tool box with well-oiled tools. On the job you could reach into your tool box and choose one to fit the specific task at hand. Good advice for any profession.

▪ CRANIAL–SACRAL THERAPY

Cranial–sacral therapy was originally an osteopathic system, based on the work done by William Sutherland, DO, in the 1940s. It works subtly on the rhythms of the dura mater, brain, spinal cord, and cerebrospinal fluid. The rhythm is palpable throughout the body at a rate of 8 to 12 cycles per minute and is used to assess and treat the body for conditions like pain, joint restrictions, fascial restriction, and unwanted patterns of posture. The theory is that restrictions in the cranial–sacral system, a semi-closed hydraulic system, will produce dysfunction in the central nervous system that is contained within this cranial–sacral system. Trauma and postural dysfunctions can cause restrictions.

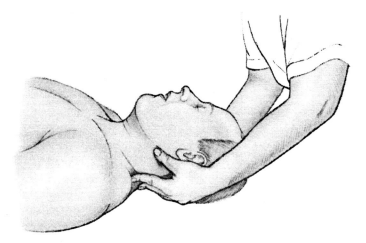

FIGURE 8–1. Cranial–sacral hold. Palpation of the atlas and occiput region to determine stress patterns and cranial–sacral fluid rhythms.

Assessment and therapeutic moves are made by holding body parts, such as a bone of the skull, bilaterally, and "listening" to the rhythms as the body moves. Assessment is made and then, by holding the skull or other part into a flexion position and stopping the system (stillpoint), the built-up pressure can gently correct any restrictions felt (Upledger & Jon, 1983) See Figure 8–1 for the correct cranial–sacral holding position.

Training is critical for this work. Good anatomical knowledge of the skull and the cranial–sacral system is required as well as good sensitivity in the hands, as the pressure used is light (5 grams). It is a restful technique for both the client and the therapist and is noninvasive. However, it creates fundamental changes when done correctly.

■ CONNECTIVE TISSUE THERAPIES OR FASCIAL TECHNIQUES

Connective tissue therapies encompass several bodies of knowledge having to do with softening connective tissue, rehydrating it, and remolding it. This is done by spreading the tissue, pulling or stretching it, and creating motion where tissues were stuck from skin rolling and fingertip stroking. Connective tissue stretching usually means taking the tissue to its point of resistance and then stretching it. Often done across fibers, this type of work can be performed subtly as in cranial–sacral therapy or as deeply as doing cross-fiber frictioning as conceived by James Cyriax.

Deep transverse frictioning is often used in sports massage and in rehabilitative massage around joints, on the musculoskeletal connections of ligaments and tendons. It results in the restructuring of the connective tissue, allows for better circulation in the area, and produces a temporary analgesia. Positioning of the muscles for the proper frictioning of the lesion is important. Also, proper rehabilitation after the massage is essential. A broadening contraction is required. The client relaxes the muscle and then contracts the muscle as far as it will go after initial work is completed.

A modified version locates a small area for friction. The muscle is placed in a relaxed position, and friction is applied transversely, against the grain of the fibers.

Elizabeth Dicke, a German physical therapist, has been credited with developing connective tissue massage in 1929. The therapy is called Bindegewebsmassage and is still taught in Europe today. Other systems have the same goal of softening layers of fascia, sometimes called ground substances, and/or inducing small inflammations that will aid in restructuring of connective tissue; they include myofascial release and others connected to postural alignment and neuromuscular therapies.

One manner in which fascial restriction is palpated in myofascial release is as follows. One hand stabilizes the tissue. The other hand pulls or pushes the tissue in the direction of the restriction. Twisting, kneading, and compression may also be applied in the direction of the restriction and can release the barrier. This style of bodywork demands more training than can be given here. Many of the modalities mentioned here are taught in the United States and Canada.

▪ FASCIAL KINETICS (BOWEN TECHNIQUE)

The Bowen form of fascial release was devised in Australia by a layperson who found that if certain points were worked in an arc of the area in a certain way, the fascia layers released and the connective tissue softened. See Figure 8–2 for a simple upper back routine.

▪ MANUAL LYMPHATIC DRAINAGE MASSAGE OR VODDER LYMPH DRAINAGE

Manual lymphatic drainage is a specific therapeutic treatment designed to reduce edema and to encourage lymphatic drainage. Edema resulting from trauma or connective tissue restrictions such as postsurgical scarring can be reduced by using light, repetitive strokes that pump the lymph through the superficial lymphatic capillaries.

The techniques are applied centripetally (towards the heart), rhythmically at proximal lymph nodes, and in overlapping strokes distally towards the edemic site. Very light pressure is used in this gliding stroke so as not to collapse the superficial lymphatic capillaries. Each stroke is repeated 5 to 7 times in order to pump the lymphatic fluid. The direction of the strokes is to the drainage points.

A pumping compression stroke is used in the beginning on the lymph nodes proximal to the edemic site. The palmar surfaces of the hands are used on larger areas to create stationary circles that spiral into the tissue and out again. In this way the edema is moved proximally. Once the site has decreased in size, the distal tissue can be treated. See Figure 8–3 for pumping strokes for lymphatic drainage.

If the therapist wishes to use this technique with Swedish massage, the manual lymph drainage should be done first. Regular Swedish massage will collapse the superficial lymphatic capillaries. Even with Swedish massage done afterwards, some

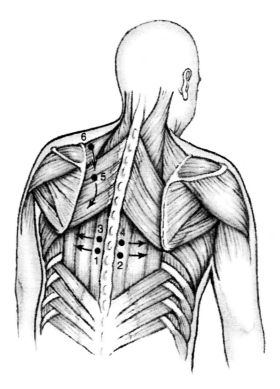

FIGURE 8–2. Fascial Kinetics (Bowen system). Various points are held or moved, sometimes in connection with breath work. In this example, points 1 to 4 are moved laterally and held through a breath and then moved over the erector spinae muscle. Repeat on the other side. A waiting period of 2 minutes follows, and then point 5 is drawn in a semicircle medially and then laterally. Point 6 is drawn back over inferior border of levator scapula. Repeat on other side of body. Repeat sequence again.

time (at least 20 minutes) should intervene between the two treatments. These techniques are slow to perform. Doing one limb can take up to 20 minutes alone.

The physiological effects of lymphatic drainage created by the toxin overload is that of feeling massage overload—generally not quite yourself. Other modalities may sometimes create the same effect.

In normal activity, exercise and deep breathing are responsible for draining the lymphatic system. When one or more of these are stopped, the lymphatic system becomes sluggish and does not work properly. Proper treatment with lymphatic drainage techniques can have an effect on the immune system.

This set of techniques was first developed by Emil Vodder, a German doctor who lived in Denmark in the 1930s. Today an Austrian Institute still teaches the techniques and has brought it to the United States and Canada. These techniques involve specialized movements and massage therapists must be properly trained to perform them correctly.

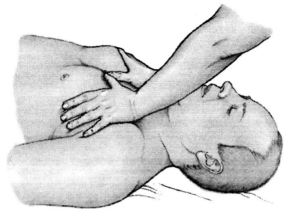

Supine

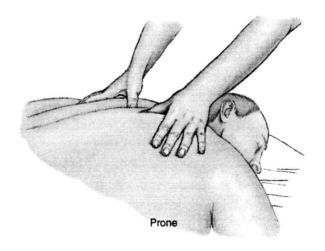

Prone

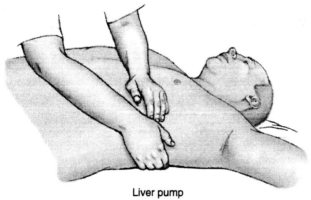

Liver pump

FIGURE 8–3. Lymphatic pumping manipulation. Pumping the lymphatic drainage system enhances the flow of lymph through the entire system (20 times per minute). May be repeated.

▪ MUSCLE ENERGY TECHNIQUES

Muscle energy techniques (METs) are a group of techniques that have been around since the 1950s. Originally from osteopathic medicine and physiotherapy, MET uses active muscular relaxation technique and is known for its gentle qualities. Earlier proprioceptive neuromuscular facilitation (PNF) used isometric exercise, strong muscular contractions, and rotation of joints to achieve the objectives.

METs are used to treat trigger points, myofascial dysfunction, and joint dysfunction. MET methods are varied but the aim is to have isometric contraction (no movement), producing a physiological–neurological response. This produces postisometric relaxation through the influence of the Golgi tendon organs or to the muscle antagonist, which produces reciprocal inhibition to its antagonist. The therapist can match the client's effort to contract the muscle in question, can exceed the client's effort, or partially match the client's effort (Chaitow, 1996b).

Many variations occur. Sometimes the antagonist muscle is used, sometimes the agonist. Sometimes the starting place of the contraction is different—at the beginning of restriction, or midway between the relaxed state and the fully stretched state.

Positioning of the muscle is often important to achieve the desired effect. The contractions are done slowly, with no jerking motions to the target muscles. (See Box 8–1 for types of muscle contractions.) Hypertonic muscles that are shortened and seem incapable of returning to their normal resting length respond well to these methods. Variations of muscle energy techniques include the following (Chaitow, 1996c).

These techniques will be described in the sections that follow:

Contract and relax or tense and relax.
Antagonist contract.

BOX 8–1   TYPES OF MUSCLE CONTRACTIONS

- *Isometric Contractions.* No movement occurs. The force of the movement of the muscle by the client is equally matched by the therapist. The distance between origin and insertion of the muscle stays constant.
- *Isotonic Contractions.* Restricted movement occurs as the force of the movement of the muscle by the client is not quite matched by the therapist. Both origin and insertion of the muscle are moved.
- *Isokinetic Contractions.* Partial resistance is offered by the therapist to the client's full range-of-motion movements at maximum strength.

Contract, relax, and contract the opposite.
Positional release/strain–counterstrain, and facilitated positional release.
Pulsed muscle energy procedures.
Integrated neuromuscular inhibition.
Chill and stretch or spray and stretch.

Contract and Relax or Tense and Relax

The contract and relax technique works on the theory that as soon as a muscle relaxes, and the muscle is then inhibited, it will relax further.

1. Position the limb so the target muscle is comfortable and lengthened.
2. Support the limb and have the client contract against resistance for 5 to 10 seconds; 30 to 50 percent contraction is good. If the client is in pain, try antagonist contraction.
3. Have the client relax muscle.
4. Move the muscle into stretch position to the point of resistance. After a short rest, repeat.
5. Back off and repeat 3 to 5 times.

Antagonist Contraction

Antagonist contraction works on the process known as **reciprocal inhibition.** When a muscle is acting on a joint, the antagonist muscle is reflexively inhibited (Fig. 8–4).

1. Position the limb so the target muscle is comfortable and lengthened.
2. Support the limb and have the client continue to stretch the muscle. Resist movement for a few seconds and then allow it to continue. If in pain, do not continue.
3. After 10 seconds, have the client relax muscle.
4. Resume stretch until resistance is felt.

Contract, Relax, and Contract the Opposite

The contract, relax, and contract the opposite technique combines the previous two techniques and was devised by Dr. Lawrence Jones.

1. Position the limb so the target muscle is comfortable but lengthened.
2. Support the limb and have the client contract the target muscle isometrically. Resistance is applied by the therapist for 5 to 10 seconds.
3. Have the client relax. Contract the opposite muscle; the limb moves into the direction of stretch. The therapist may assist.
4. Allow a short rest and then repeat.

The technique is useful on recent strains.

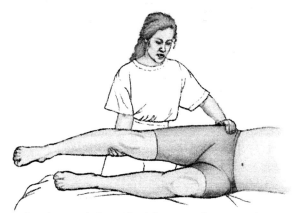

Isolate the muscle by putting it into a passive contraction.
Move origin and insertion of muscle together to do this.

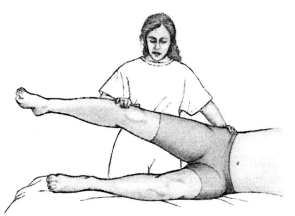

Stop contraction, bring muscle into a lengthened state,
stopping at resistance.

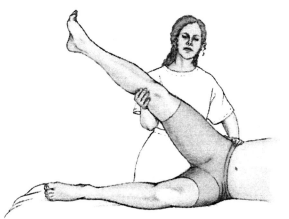

Place muscle into contraction again.
Repeat until normal full resting length is obtained.

FIGURE 8–4. Reciprocal inhibition technique.

Positional Release/Strain–Counterstrain and Facilitated Positional Release

Positional release or the strain–counterstrain technique locates tender points, usually in the antagonist muscle. The body part is then moved into the direction of ease. The body maintains this position for 30 seconds to 1 minute until a change is felt. Slowly the body is returned to a neutral point. The treatment can be repeated several times until the full normal resting length is secured. This technique is good to use for muscle spasms (Fig. 8–5).

Facilitated positional release is a variation on the strain–counterstrain method (Fig. 8–6). The distressed area is positioned into the direction of its greatest freedom of movement. One of the therapist's hands "listens" to the area while the other hand maintains medium pressure for 5 seconds. Another method holds light pressure on the area and drags the tissue (Chaitow, 1996c).

Pulsed Muscle Energy Procedures

Pulsed muscle energy procedures use the barrier of the muscle and small resisted contractions (2 per second), which mechanically pumps. It also uses contract and relax and reciprocal inhibitions.

1. Isolate the muscle into a passive contraction.
2. Apply counterpressure.
3. Have the client rapidly contract muscle in small movements. Do twenty repetitions.
4. Slowly lengthen the muscle. Repeat until full normal resting length is obtained.

All of these techniques work because the body is repositioned into the original strain. This allows the muscle proprioceptors to reset and stop firing pain and danger signals.

Integrated Neuromuscular Inhibition

With integrated neuromuscular inhibition (INIT), the position of ease is maintained while ischaemic compression is applied. An isometric contraction into the tissue is added and held for 7 to 10 seconds and then stretching is added (Chaitow, 1996a).

Chill and Stretch or Spray and Stretch

Chill and stretch has replaced spray and stretch technique due to the environmental harm caused by a vapocoolant that contributes to ozone depletion. Chilling and stretching an area containing a trigger point helps to deactivate the abnormal neurological behavior of the site (Fig. 8–7). The brief interruption of the pain–spasm–pain cycle may be sufficient to remove the trigger points (Travell, 1983).

Ice, or a cold drink can frozen and rolled over the tissue, will often reduce or eliminate the trigger point from the area. The ice or cold can is swept over the area in one direction only and is swept over the area again after a few seconds. Passive stretch may follow the procedures. Simple exercises can be added for self-help care with the client using gentle heat at home.

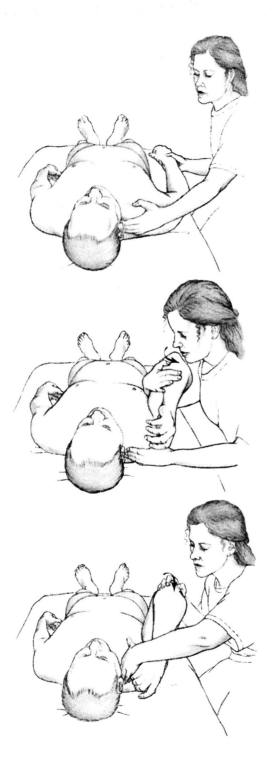

A tender spot is identified
by the therapist in the client's
supraspinatus muscle.
(left hand)

By positioning the client's
arm the tender spot begins
to ease.

A greater degree of ease is
found and the position is
held for 20 to 60 seconds.

FIGURE 8–5. Strain–counterstrain positional release techniques.

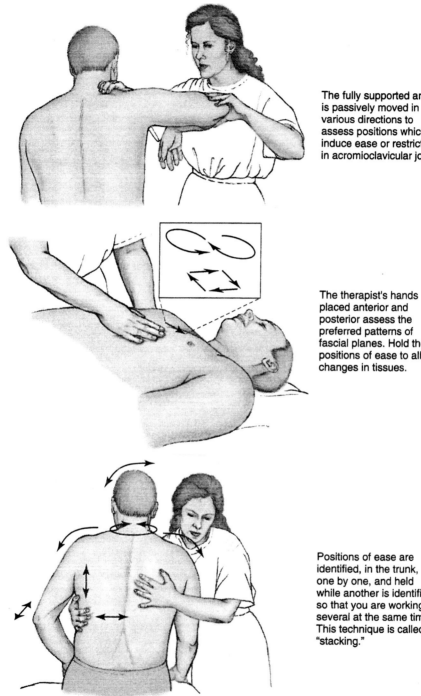

The fully supported arm is passively moved in various directions to assess positions which induce ease or restriction in acromioclavicular joint.

The therapist's hands placed anterior and posterior assess the preferred patterns of fascial planes. Hold the positions of ease to allow changes in tissues.

Positions of ease are identified, in the trunk, one by one, and held while another is identified, so that you are working on several at the same time. This technique is called "stacking."

FIGURE 8–6. Facilitated positional release.

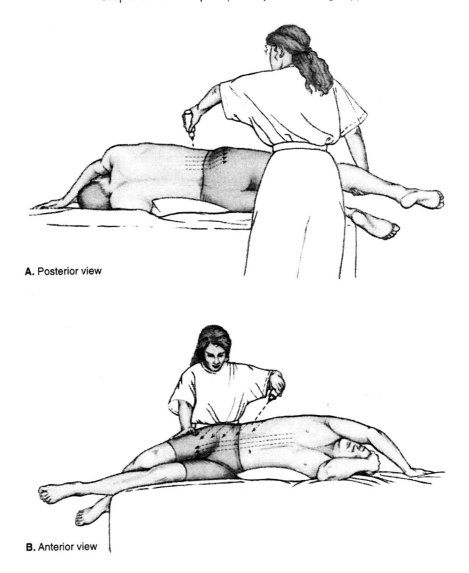

A. Posterior view

B. Anterior view

FIGURE 8–7. Chill and stretch or spray and stretch technique used on trigger points. The client stretches muscle fibers of quadratus lumborum with trigger points, while the therapist uses a vapocoolant spray or ice to spray or cool the area in a fan-like pattern.

▪ MYOFASCIAL TECHNIQUES

Although myofascial techniques are connective tissue techniques, they are treated here separately because they are connected with the whole body. The theories are based on body changes created by working on the crystalline substance of fasciae, which in turn changes the **piezoelectric current** (an electrical, chemical, and magnetic communication system in the tissue that keeps the tissue soft). This system of fasciae acts in response to stress and strain. Another component of connective tissue is the **ground substance,** a gel-like substance containing collagen fibers and fibroblasts (Fig. 8–8). The function of this ground substance is to diffuse nutrients and wastes and act as a mechanical barrier to invading bacteria. With trauma or injury, dehydration of this ground substance occurs. The fibers crowd and begin to bind together, forming hard, tough tissue that cannot move. The tissue becomes stuck to surrounding tissue and organs.

Several techniques are used to soften the tissues and allow movement. There is a myofascial component in several systems: Rolfing®, myofascial release, SOMA (Greek word meaning body and mind), and Neuromuscular Integration and Structural Alignment (NISA).

The strokes used in myofascial techniques include a spreading technique, which takes the tissue to the restriction and then spreads the multidimensional fascia fibers. Lift or scoop the tissue up as you begin to work it with your entry at a 90-degree angle. Wait for the tissue to melt, or push through the barrier if you think it will melt. A gliding stroke can be applied to help stretch the tissue. When a soft-

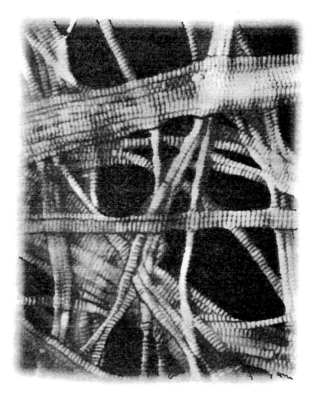

FIGURE 8–8. A fascia ground substance showing web-like collagen fibers in a gel-like substance.

ening occurs, stop working in that area. When tissue seems unresponsive, ask the client to move the stuck area, or ask for deeper breathing in the area you are working. See Figure 8–9 for myofascial release techniques.

Another muscle energy technique combining applied kinesiology, neural lymphatic massage points, and neurovascular holding points is Touch for Health. See Appendix F for more information.

▪ NEUROMUSCULAR TECHNIQUES

The goal of neuromuscular techniques is to increase mobility and reduce pain, fatigue, depression, and stress. Soft tissue injuries are identified and assessed and then normalized to proper function. In this way the pain cycle (Chap. 3) is broken and the tissue is encouraged to improve function. Neuromuscular therapy addresses trigger points, and acupuncture points may be used (Fig. 8–10). Postural distortions are addressed and sometimes the therapy is combined with other modalities (Chaitow, 1996a). Some of the strokes used are the following:

- *Gliding.* Usually using the thumb, light pressure is employed to assess and deeper pressure used later to stretch the fascia and release adhesions.
- *Compression.* Pressure is held on painful spots and trigger points, but always below the client's pain threshold. Pressure is generally held 8 to 12 seconds. Often a T-bar can be used on deep trigger points (Fig. 8–11).
- *Skin rolling.* The skin is picked up and rolled to separate the various layers.
- *Stretching.* Stretching is done after tissue is loosened. The muscle and connective tissue involved need to achieve their normal resting length, and this is done with active and passive stretching. Muscle energy techniques may also be used. Regular exercise may be used as client self-care if needed.

This technique was developed in England by Dr. Stanley Lief in the 1930s, with his cousin, Boris Chaitow. Paul St. John has popularized the method and teaches a whole body approach through a series of seminars around the country. Other systems (such as NISA) incorporate the technique. Visceral techniques are also taught, using neuromuscular and fascial techniques to manipulate the organs of the body.

Often fascial and neuromuscular restrictions create postural and structural problems. By clearly understanding the underlying anatomy and by using these techniques, we can alleviate many structural problems for our clients. More training is needed so that the techniques may be used properly. Several other techniques are categorized as "neuromuscular"—Trager®, myotherapy, proprioceptive neuromuscular facilitation (PNF), reflexology, and trigger points, to name a few.

Orthobionomy

Orthobionomy was developed by an English osteopath named Arthur Lincoln Pauls after he had read of the work of Dr. Lawrence Jones. It is based on the body's

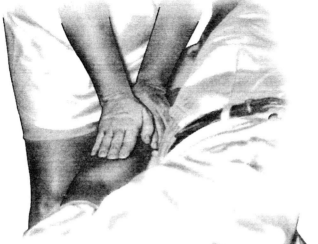

A

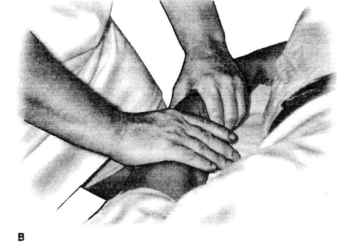

B

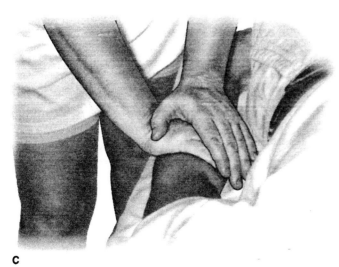

C

FIGURE 8–9. Myofascial release technique. **A.** One hand stabilizes tissue while the other hand pulls or pushes tissue in the direction of the restriction. **B.** Use twisting, kneading, and compression to release barrier. **C.** Compression.

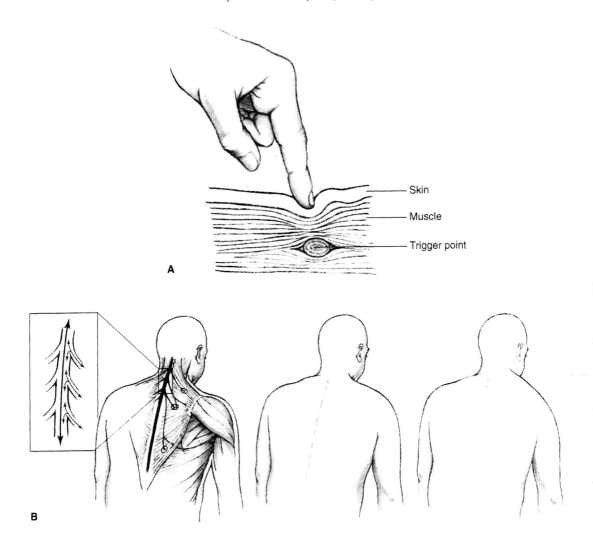

FIGURE 8–10. A. Trigger points and trigger point evolvement in dysfunctional fibrotic tissue. **B.** Example of trigger point evolvement. The dysfunctional fibrotic state increases as does the tone of the trigger point.

self-correcting reflexes. Orthobionomy seeks to restore the body's natural understanding by moving the body slowly into and through those places where fear or habit have taken it. Blocked vital energy, pain, and restricted movement are reduced or eliminated.

Passive positioning methods are used to relax muscles and ligaments. Trigger points and passive joint movements are addressed. Often mental and emotional release accompanies the work due to its gentle nature. Self-healing is sought through improved circulation and energy flow (Feltman, 1989).

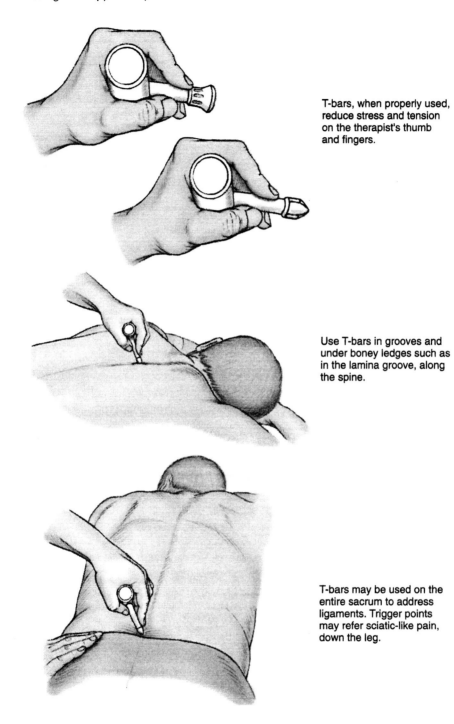

T-bars, when properly used, reduce stress and tension on the therapist's thumb and fingers.

Use T-bars in grooves and under boney ledges such as in the lamina groove, along the spine.

T-bars may be used on the entire sacrum to address ligaments. Trigger points may refer sciatic-like pain, down the leg.

FIGURE 8–11. Use of T-bars.

Reflexology or Zone Therapy

Reflexology stimulates the body's healing by stimulating specific points on the feet that correspond to and affect organs and other distant parts of the body. Reflexology operates on the theory that every part of the body refers to a point on the hands, feet, and ears. By applying pressure to the point on the feet, the therapist can effect certain changes. See Figures 8–12 to 8–14 for reflexology points. Another theory is the 10-zone theory, which states that there are 10 zones running from the top of the head to the feet. The specific points stimulated on the feet and hands run through these zones. These therapies improve circulation and the elimination of wastes and reduce stress.

Reflexology has an advantage when a person cannot get on a table or does not want to remove clothing. When a body part other than the feet is injured, it is generally unwise to work the injured area; working on the feet is an indirect way to work on the injury.

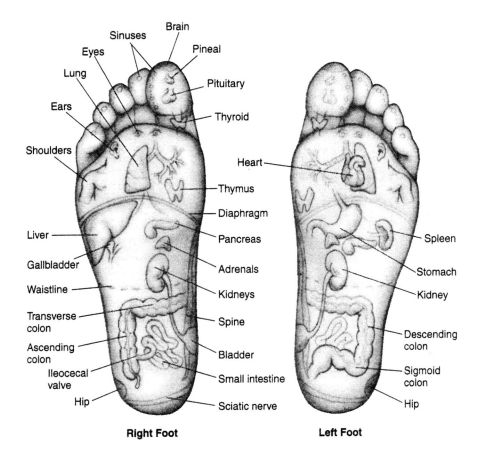

FIGURE 8–12. Foot reflexology diagram.

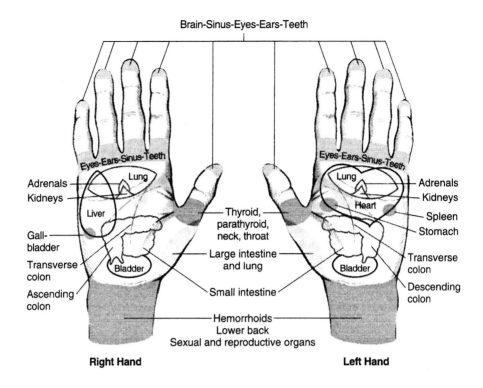

FIGURE 8–13. Hand reflexology diagram.

Reflexologists do not diagnose or claim to cure illnesses. Soreness in a reflex point on the feet or hands indicates an imbalance, which can be temporary or chronic. Very tender or painful areas should be checked by a physician. Be sure as a therapist that you master this technique before working on the public. Charts are available that show the points on the foot and their corresponding body parts (Kunz & Kunz, 1982).

Trigger Points or Myofascial Therapy

The trigger point technique has been made popular by a Miami physician, Janet Travell. While it is incorporated in many treatment approaches, Dr. Travell's work and Bonnie Prudden's myotherapy, both remain very popular. Dr. Leon Chaitow also uses the technique in his work.

Although not connected to the Oriental style of acupressure treatment, this therapy works on the theory that trigger points are small areas of hypertonicity or sensitivity within muscles located near motor nerve points. Once aggravated by stress and other irritants in a body, they can fire and set off contractions in muscle

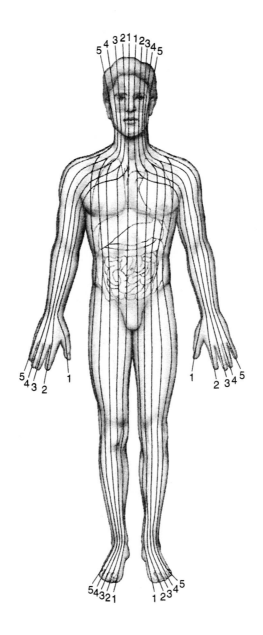

FIGURE 8–14. Zones of the body as used in reflexology.

bundle fibers and subsequently activate an entire muscle. Referred pain from this site can radiate out to a larger area of the body. Dr. Travell's books give these patterns of referred pain, the points themselves, and the methods of direct pressuring, dry needling, acupuncture, or chill and stretch as suggested treatments. All treatment should be done below the client's pain threshold. Other methods used are similar to those described in the "Neuromuscular Techniques" section earlier in the chapter. Trigger point work is intensive and may only be tolerated for a short time by the client (15 to 30 minutes).

Once a trigger point is found, direct pressure is added, usually by the therapist's thumb, and then stretching is done to eliminate the point. The belly of the muscle is first pushed together to affect the spindle cells; if that is not successful, muscle fibers in the belly are separated towards the tendons. Direct pressure against a hard underlying structure may be accomplished, or a pinching or squeezing pressure may be done when the surrounding tissue is soft. The time of applied pressure is usually 8 to 10 seconds, with the therapist gradually building pressure and stopping when the client or therapist feels a release. Variable pressure is suggested by some to avoid further injury. Deep cross-fiber friction may also be used, especially if surrounding tissue is stuck. It is believed that gradual lengthening to reset the normal resting length of the neuromuscular mechanism of the muscle, and stretching to elongate shortened connective tissue of the treated muscle, is necessary for the treatment to maintain normalcy. Moist heat and rest are suggested after treatment.

Traditionally, only physician-referred clients sought myotherapists; but many massage therapists use the term "myotherapy" and treat trigger points. Some therapists use T-bars and "bilos" (short wooden shafts) to get at deep trigger points. Otherwise, the thumb, fingers, or elbows are used (Travell & Simons, 1983). See Figure 8–15 for trigger points of the back.

Trager® Technique

The Trager® technique's approach is through communication to the muscles and the joints as well as gentle range-of-motion movements accomplished through gentle rocking and shaking. The body is coaxed into free movement (Fig. 8–16).

Dr. Milton Trager is responsible for this modality, which is based on patterns of body posture and body compensations held in the mind. Releasing those patterns in the mind, in his view, will improve all systems of the body.

> *My work is really a philosophy, not bodywork or massage. Its goal is to bring people into a state of hook-up, feeling connected to a vibratory force, without which you're no place. If we all had hook-up, there would be no wars (Feltman, Hands-on Healing, p. 326).*

A self-help component for both therapist and client is the "mentastics" exercises, which use gravity and the body's own weight to move body parts (Feltman, 1989).

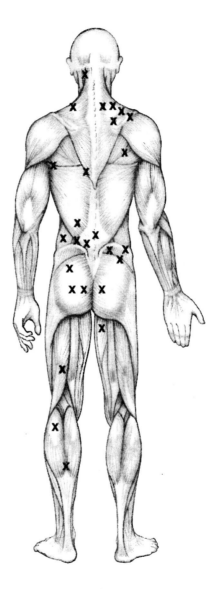

FIGURE 8–15. Prominent trigger points of the back.

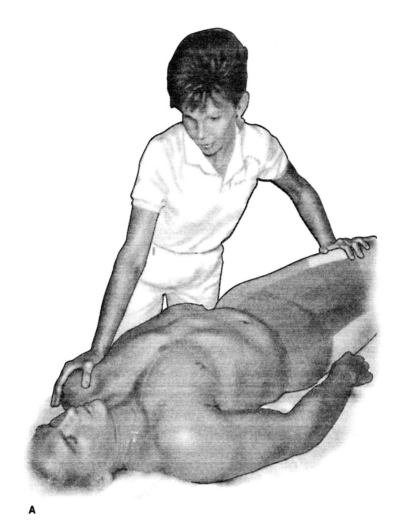

A

FIGURE 8–16. The Trager® approach. **A.** Therapist stretches the hip rotators and sacral attachments by flexing the leg and moving it across the body in a "leg around" movement. *(Continued)*

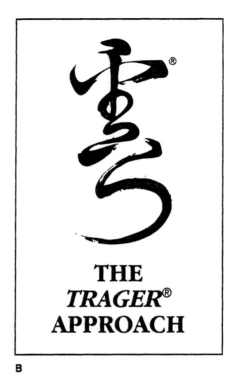

B

FIGURE 8–16 (cont.). The Trager® approach. **B.** Mind–body approach logo.

▪ ORIENTAL THERAPIES

Eastern style therapies are many and varied and are becoming very popular in the West. A few of the theories underlying these systems of massage will be given here, followed by a quick summary of Oriental-style massage. The usual contraindications apply to Oriental massage.

Yin and **yang,** the opposite aspects of matter and phenomena in nature, are interdependent and complementary. Everything in the universe has yin and yang characteristics. When these are balanced in the human body as well as in nature, perfect balance exists.

Chi (qi, ki) is the vital energy that activates life. It nourishes and protects the body. Chi and the blood go together. If the flow of blood is interrupted, both chi and the blood stagnate in their channels, causing pain and eventually dysfunction (Shen, 1996). See Figure 8–17 for diagrams showing energy channels in the body.

A system of channels through which chi flows consists of 12 regular channels called **meridians** or **meridian lines** and 2 extra channels. The channels are distributed symmetrically on both sides of the body and are connected to each other to form a continuous circuit. Each of the 12 regular channels connects with one of the

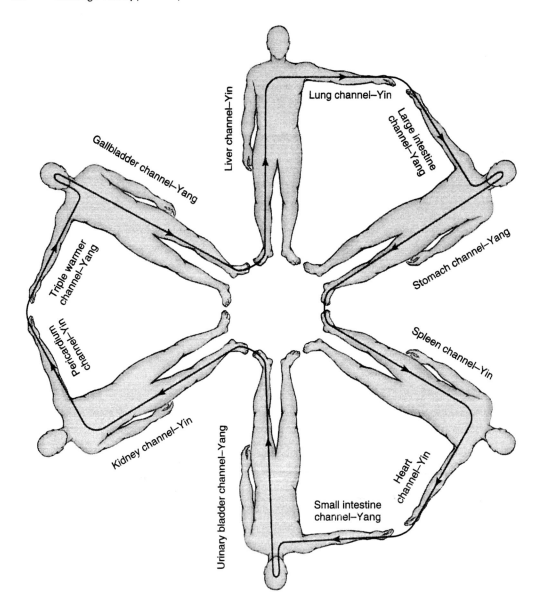

FIGURE 8–17. Yin and yang channels diagram.

internal organs, follows a course along either leg or arm, and is associated with either yin or yang. The yin channels flow upwards on the inside surfaces of the front of the body while the yang channels flow downward on the outer surfaces of the back of the body. The yin channels converge in the abdomen, and the yang channels in the head region. Each channel meets its paired channel at either the hand or the foot (Fig. 8–18).

The association between symptoms and channel disturbance forms the basis for pain relief massage treatments. Carefully chosen acupoints are massaged, and pain is relieved. The channels are open, the blood and chi can flow through, yin and yang are balanced, and pain is resolved. See Figure 8–19 for the acupoints along the gallbladder meridian. Six basic techniques are used on the acupoints:

- Light pressure to stroke and rub.
- Rubbing and kneading.
- Small rotations by the thumb.
- Pinching, squeezing, and kneading.
- Vibration.
- Tapping.

Another theory related to the organs is the five-element theory. The organs are divided into five categories, relating to the five elements.

Amna (Amma) massage is originally Chinese, but migrated through Korea to Japan over 1500 years ago. Amma generally works away from the heart, on over 100 acupoints in the body. It is done over clothing or a towel and all 12 meridian lines are worked (Sohn & Einando, 1988).

Chinese massage is based on prevention rather than on cure. In Peijian Shen's book *Massage for Pain Relief*, a client self-help massage is illustrated as well as a full body massage routine. Strokes are listed with their Chinese names (Shen, 1996).

- Pressing—an
- Pushing—tui
- Rubbing—Mo
- Kneading—ron
- Pinching—qia
- Squeezing—na
- Wiping—moz

Acupuncture and Acupressure

A branch of Chinese medicine, **acupuncture** is an ancient system of inserting thin needles along meridian lines in the body to correspond with body parts and functions (**tsubos**) and to stimulate and control the chi or life force. The purpose is to stabilize the body and create homeostasis. **Acupressure** is a modification of this system, devised in the Western world. The effects of both systems are well known and deserve our attention in massage. The strokes used in acupressure are basically

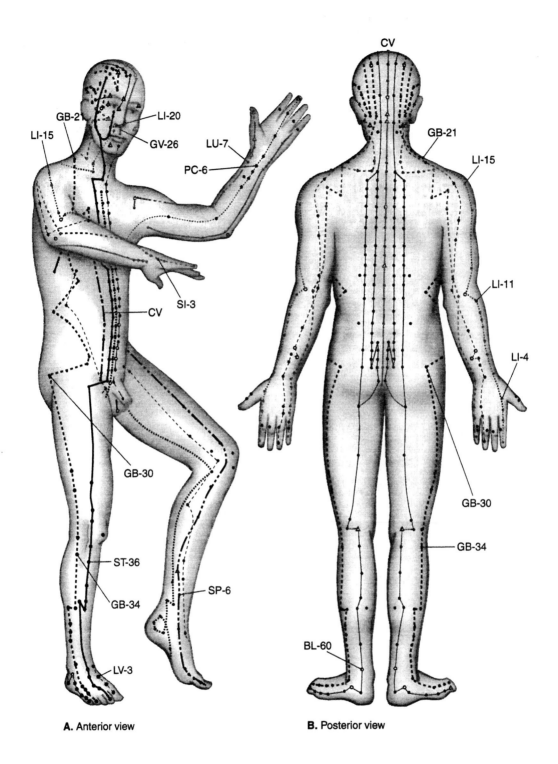

FIGURE 8–18. Energy channels (meridians). Each channel connects to an internal organ, runs along an arm or leg, and is considered yin or yang energy. Yin energy travels upward, yang energy travels downward. *(Continued)*

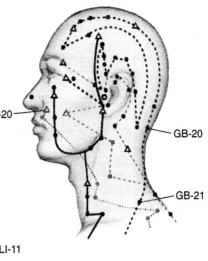

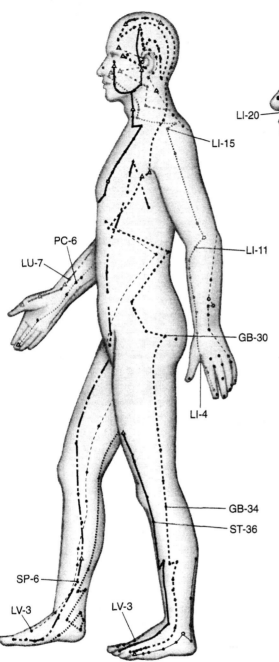

LI-20

GB-20

GB-21

LI-15

PC-6

LU-7

LI-11

GB-30

LI-4

Yin and yang channels

Stomach–Yang	ST
Gallbladder–Yang	GB
Kidney–Yin	KI
Spleen–Yin	SP
Governing Vessel	GV
Heart–Yin	HT
Small Intestine–Yang	SI
Large Intestine–Yang	LI
Lung–Yin	LU
Urinary bladder–Yang	BL
Liver–Yin	LV
Triple Warmer–Yang	TW
Pericardium	PC
Conception Vessel	CV

GB-34

ST-36

SP-6

LV-3

LV-3

C. Lateral view

FIGURE 8–18 (cont.).

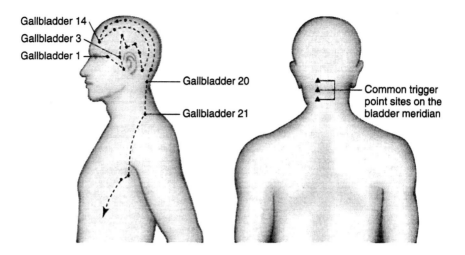

FIGURE 8–19. Trigger point sites along the gallbladder meridian.

touching a point, adding pressure to the point, and rubbing the point. The point is usually held between 3 and 10 seconds. Well-developed muscles might take pressure up to 2 minutes.

Acupressure is generally thought to be best suited to treating aches and pains, stress, menstrual cramps, asthma, and arthritis. Acupuncture is generally thought to be better at treating chronic or severe pain and is used in Asia for surgery anaesthesia. In many states in the United States, a license separate from a massage license is needed to practice acupuncture. Check with your state department of regulations.

Do-in

Do-in (pronounced "dough-in") is an exercise practice introduced into the United States by Michio Kusho Cushion associated with the publication of the *East West Journal.* The exercise practices are based on the theory of human adaptation to the natural environment. Their purpose is to produce physical health and spiritual harmony with the universe.

The do-in exercises are self-help techniques that often resemble yoga postures. They are designed to work with the body's energy meridians (Feltman, 1989).

Shiatsu

A Japanese system of acupressure, shiatsu also works on the tsubos or acupuncture points, though it does not correspond completely with the Chinese method. Pressure is exerted on the points with the pads of the finger or thumb for 2 to 5 seconds or more, depending on the area. Some practitioners use electrical stimulation instead of the hands. Routines have been devised for the whole body and to reduce

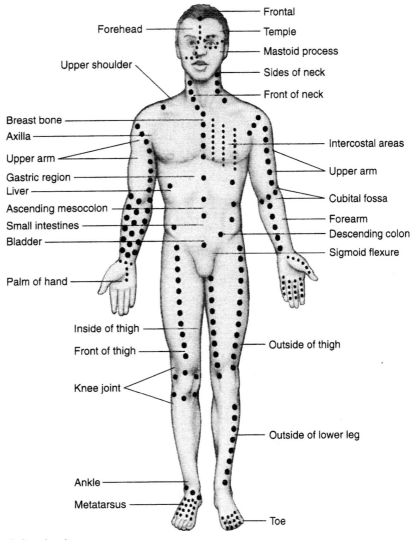

A. Anterior view

FIGURE 8–20. Pressure points. *(Continued)*

certain common symptoms. They can be done on a table or a floor mat. See Figure 8–20 for pressure points to be massaged in shiatsu. Ohashi, the founder of the Ohashi Institute, states that "shiatsu is an integral part of maintaining health along with meditation, diet and exercise." The purpose of shiatsu is to increase circulation and restore the energetic system of the body (Fig. 8–21). Shiatsu is taught in several schools in the United States and Canada. See Appendix E for a basic shiatsu routine.

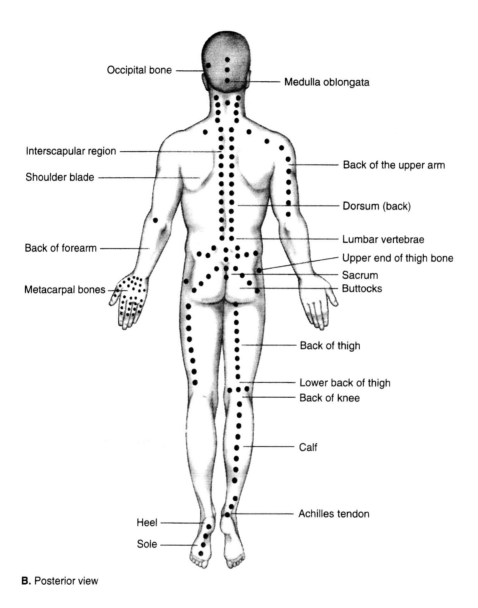

Occipital bone

Medulla oblongata

Interscapular region

Back of the upper arm

Shoulder blade

Dorsum (back)

Lumbar vertebrae

Back of forearm

Upper end of thigh bone

Sacrum

Metacarpal bones

Buttocks

Back of thigh

Lower back of thigh

Back of knee

Calf

Achilles tendon

Heel

Sole

B. Posterior view

FIGURE 8–20 (cont.). Pressure points.

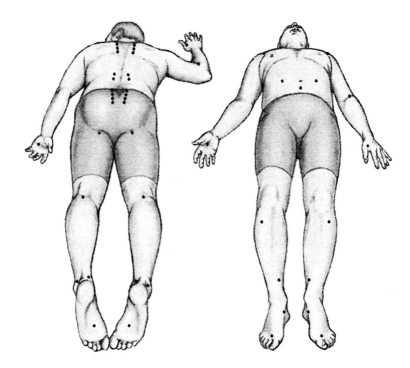

FIGURE 8–21. Basic shiatsu routine. Work on floormat.

Sometimes, instead of using fingers, hands, elbows, or feet to create pressure on a certain point, herbs are burned over the point (**moxibustion**). The herb moxa, which is the down that grows on the underside of *Artemisia vulgaris* or mugwort, is pinched into a cone, which is placed on the skin and ignited. The herb is meant to release its drawing powers to draw inflammation to the surface (Fig. 8–22). A thin slice of ginger root may be placed between it and the skin. The smoldering herb has a pungent odor (Culpepper).

To learn acupressure, acupuncture, or shiatsu, it is necessary to study with a skilled teacher. The history and theory of the system is an integral part of learning the actual points (tsubos). Proficiency in any of these techniques takes time to develop. As stated before, acupuncture may require a separate license. For books and associations to contact for further information, see Appendix F.

Thai Massage

Thai massage is a combination of working on the meridians to open them, stretches, and massage strokes (Fig. 8–23). It is the ancient art of Thailand, still done today in the Buddhist tradition. It is becoming popular the United States. The technique is done on a floormat.

Other Oriental techniques include jin shin do, Hoshino, tuina, watsu, and Tibetan point holding.

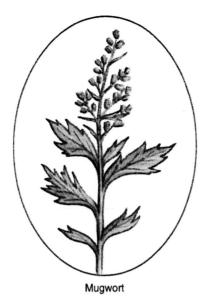

Mugwort

FIGURE 8–22. The mugwort plant (*Artemisia vulgaris*).

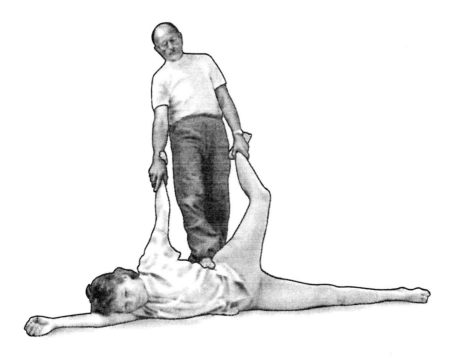

FIGURE 8–23. Thai massage. Once the meridians of the body are opened, the joints of the body are stretched.

▪ SEATED MASSAGE

In recent years, seated massage has captured the imagination of the corporate world. Many well-known businesses employ massage therapists to come to their offices regularly to perform massage on their employees using a folding massage chair. Clothes are not removed. Other businesses arrange health fairs for their employees once or twice a year, and the line waiting for a turn in the massage chair is the longest. Massages often raise the morale of employees, increase productivity, and reduce sick leave. Some employers even help pay for the sessions and use them as an incentive for their employees.

Several massage table manufacturers also produce a folding chair or a tabletop device that offers support and comfort for the client. Figure 8–24 shows a massage being done on a chair manufactured for seated massage. If you do not have a seated massage chair, the technique can also be performed with the client sitting sideways on a straightback chair or backwards with the arms, head, and shoulders positioned on a tabletop with pillows for comfort.

Usually, a seated massage is 10 to 20 minutes long and covers the back, neck, shoulders, arms, and low back. For the seated chair routine, see Appendix E.

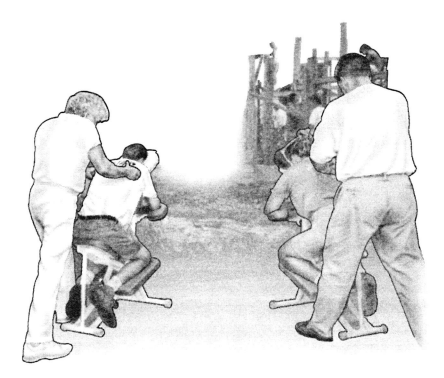

FIGURE 8–24. Seated massage.

▪ STRUCTURAL ALIGNMENT AND POSTURAL INTEGRATION TECHNIQUES

There are several types of structural alignment techniques, but all of them started with Rolfing® as developed by Dr. Ida Rolf and the Rolf Institute. The basis of Rolfing® is the alignment of the body parts through the manipulation of the fasciae. The connective tissue is affected, in turn, as are the tonus receptor mechanisms. Positional releases are sought, the reflex arc is stimulated, and once the tissue is loosened, softened, and moldable, stretching and lengthening occurs.

Various systems have developed from Rolfing®, notably Hellerwork, Neuromuscular Integration and Structural Alignment (NISA), SOMA, CORE, Looyen, and Pfrimmer. All of these align the body through a series of treatments aimed at facilitating the necessary structural corrections. See Figure 8–25 for evidence of the changes that can be effected during a series of structural alignment treatments. All

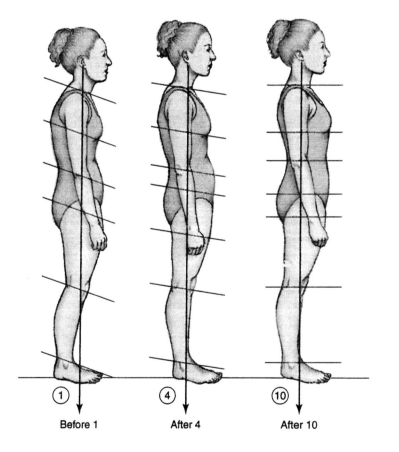

Before 1   After 4   After 10

FIGURE 8–25. Structural alignment series. Common progressive changes of body planes during a series of structural alignment treatments. Notice changes from oblique planes to horizontal planes (before 1st treatment, after 4th treatment, and after 10th treatment).

of these systems involve further training. Seminars and workshops are given across the United States and Canada.

▪ VIBRATIONAL THERAPIES OR ENERGY THERAPY

The therapies listed under this heading may seem to be less physiologically oriented than others, but they deal with a vital aspect of the human body—the life force. Although partially rooted in Eastern beliefs and theories, these modalities have been developed in the West. Modern medicine has a hard time believing in them; many people do. They are certainly part of the movement of massage and bodywork and deserve our attention. Because they can often be performed without removing clothing and when contraindications would rule out regular massage, they offer the therapist another tool to use even when massage may not be done.

Polarity Therapy

Polarity therapy is based on the theory that energy, or a vibrational field, surrounds us and runs through the body at all times. The better the current flows, the healthier the person will be. Randolph Stone, an osteopath, based this modality on ancient writings about the cosmos and on some current scientific writings

The balancing of the energies in the human body is accomplished through the use of the therapist's energy. The therapist's hands are held on the body in a resting position. Current, or energy, runs between the hands, balancing the energies. (It is similar to using booster cables on your car.) The current of energy is subtle, of course, and sometimes a light squeeze of the therapist's hands pumps the body to start change. The hands of the therapist move around the body—knees and pelvis, sides of the neck, feet and hips—balancing as they move. The sessions give the client a wonderful sense of well-being (Feltman, 1989). See Figure 8–26 for typical hand positions in polarity.

You can learn this modality on your own through books and practice. The Polarity Therapy Association does offer seminars and workshops around the country.

Aura Balancing or Stroking

Aura balancing is done by brushing or stroking the aura, an energy field felt just off the body. It is thought that many problems and diseases can be felt in the aura before they manifest in the physical body. If they can be corrected there, the body will not be subjected to them. In order to preserve health and recreate health, the auric field needs balancing.

Some theories suggest that the therapist uses his or her own energy, stored in the chakras (organ-related energy centers in the trunk), and draws the energy from the chakras through the hands to the client's body. Where energy is blocked, it is washed out; where it is undercharged, it is charged. Where it is torn or leaking, it is patched up and balanced.

It takes additional training to learn this method.

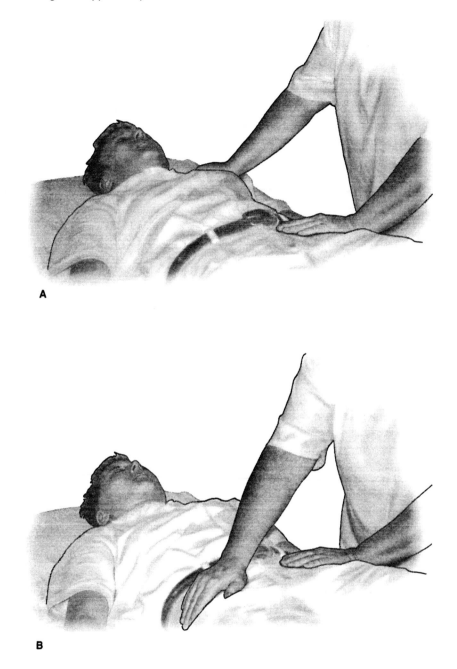

FIGURE 8–26. Polarity balancing. Typical hand positions used in polarity to balance energy. **A.** Hand position on shoulder and waist. **B.** Hand position on hips to balance joints. *(Continued)*

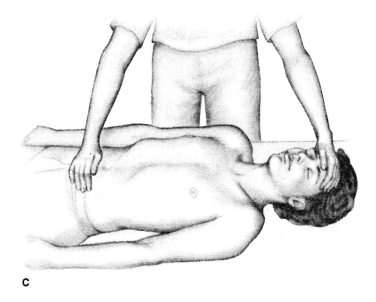

c

FIGURE 8–26 (cont.). C. Balancing out energies between head and midtorso.

Reiki

There are many variations on the technique of reiki, which has Japanese roots. They all deal with changing the energy in a person's body by laying on of hands. The purpose is to relieve the body of blockages that affect the body, emotions, and spirit. There are several steps in learning this technique and it requires a qualified teacher.

Therapeutic Touch

Therapeutic touch works just off the body and was developed by a nurse. It is used in hospitals and nursing homes and is highly effective.

Color Therapy (Chromotherapy) and Sound Therapy

The use of color and sound in therapy is not new. Historically, sound and color have been used for a long time. The Egyptians used colored liquids, set in the sun, to collect the sun's energies, much as sun tea is made today. In the medical field, sound has been used on mental health patients for decades.

It is thought that the seven colors of the spectrum are attuned to the seven tones of the musical scale. By producing the vibrations of color or sound to match the particular individual's vibration or area of the body deficient in that vibration, a vibrational change will occur and the person may be healed. Color is usually

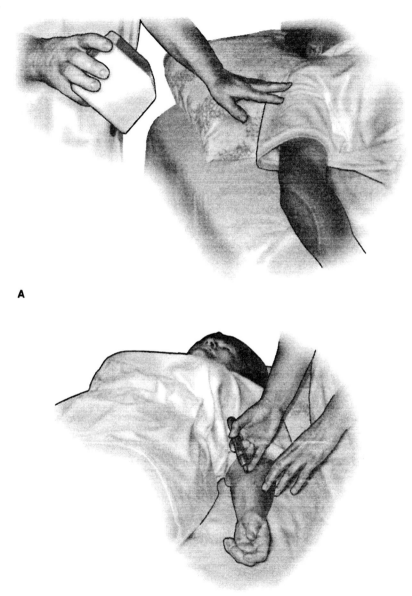

A

B

FIGURE 8–27. Use of spectrum-splitting electric light box in color therapy. **A.** Color therapy spectrum-splitting machine beams light onto the body (notice rainbow on arm). **B.** Color puncture therapy used with acupressure points directly on the skin.

produced by a small spectrum-splitting electric light box and the color may be aimed at the client or diffused into the treatment room (Fig. 8–27). In sound therapy, the chanting voice, tuning devices, and music are used to create the vibrational changes needed. Often sound therapy is used with polarity to affect the chakras or energy centers of the body.

Because many massage therapists already use music in their treatment rooms, we need to learn as much about sound therapy as we can. Research is needed in both of these areas to further their development in the massage field (Amber, 1983).

Aromatherapy

Aromatherapy combines the essential oils of flowers, herbs, woods, bark, or leaves with the lubricant generally used for massage in order to deeply penetrate the skin and provide healing for the client. The oils resemble expensive perfumes, while their properties have been known for centuries. Many oils have antiseptic effects that can protect from infection. Some have the effect of regeneration in the skin. Choose the carrier oil carefully, as the smell of each type of oil is different. See Figure 7–30 for a variety of aromatherapy products.

Many massage therapists create their own blends and have several on hand to match the client's purpose for a massage (Box 8–2). Many good books on aromatherapy discuss the properties of different oils.

Another variation is herb oil that can be made by placing herbs in a jar with almond oil and letting it sit in the sun. Shake occasionally. After 2 to 3 weeks, strain the oil through cheesecloth and muslin to filter. Refrigerate the oil when not in use (Worwood, 1996). Figure 8–28 shows different types of diffusers.

Animal Massage

Another modality gaining in popularity is massage to animals. Whether you prefer a large animal like a horse (equine massage) or small animals like the family pet, massage can be just the treatment for injury, illness, and special problems such as dysplasia, arthritis, and old age (Figs. 8–29 and 8–30). The reasons for massaging

---

BOX 8–2   QUICK AND EASY BLENDS OF OIL

- *Calming effect.* For a balancing of energy, use chamomile, lavender, orange, marjoram, and fir.
- *Tonic effect.* For a stimulating massage, use lemon, peppermint, sage, and thyme.
- *Circulation improvement.* To stimulate blood and lymph flow, use lemon, cypress, geranium, grapefruit, and thyme.
- *Pain reliever.* To ease neuralgia and muscular pain, use birch, clove, juniper, ginger, and marjoram.

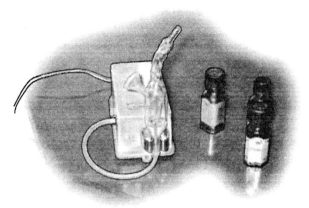

A. Aromatherapy oils or essential oils are put directly into the diffuser machine. A light mist of fragrance is directed into the air.

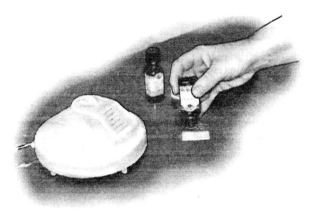

B. Aromatherapy oils or essential oils are placed on a small pad and it is placed into the machine. A light mist of fragrance is dispersed into the air.

FIGURE 8–28. Several types of diffusers. *(Continued)*

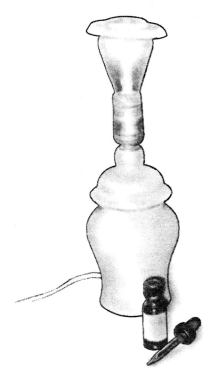

C. Aromatherapy oils or essential oils are placed on a porous ring. The lamp is turned on and heat dispenses fragrance into the room.

FIGURE 8–28 (cont.). Several types of diffusers.

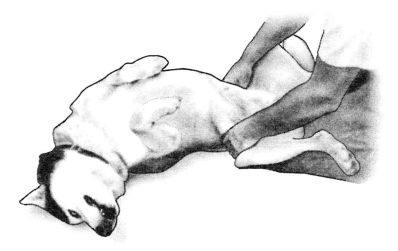

FIGURE 8–29. Massaging a highly active family pet (here an Alaskan Husky).

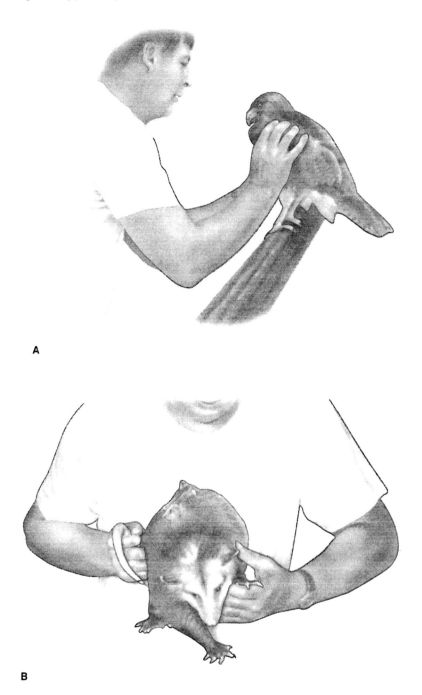

A

B

FIGURE 8–30. Injured animals receiving massage as part of their rehabilitation process. **A.** Falcon receiving massage on an injured wing. **B.** Opposum receiving massage (note the babies on her back).

animals, large or small, are the same or similar to the reasons for massaging people. Stress and tension are a part of life, whether the animal is injured or highly active. Maintaining health is also important as certain animals are expensive to own and perhaps are also a source of income for their owners.

Fortunately, many animals have anatomy and physiology similar to humans (Fig. 8–31). Thus, massage therapists are able to adapt easily to the muscles of these animals. Horses, for instance, are engaged in many kinds of activities—such as racing, hunting, dressage, playing polo, and performing—so that the sore areas are quite varied on a horse (Fig. 8–32).

Safety around large animals is an important factor. The therapist working with horses needs to be aware of their strength and potential violence if they are really hurt. Smaller animals may bite and scratch, so knowing your animal before you endeavor to massage it is a must.

Several certification programs around the country advertise in massage journals. Be certain that you know what the training will entail before you sign up for the program. Job opportunities are numerous, but as with massage therapy for people, your ability and training are very important in the job market. Specializing in the horse and the rider together gives the therapist a twofold client base.

The main originator of equine massage therapy is Jack Meagher.

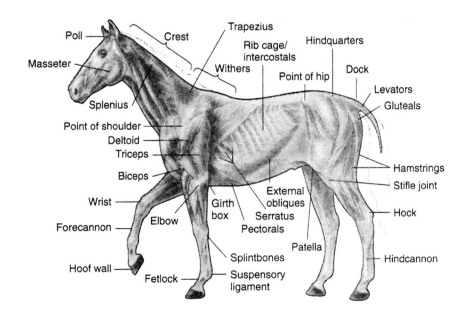

FIGURE 8–31. Chart of horse anatomy. Notice the similarities to human anatomy. The names of some muscles are the same (trapezius, hamstrings, serratus). Also notice some of the differences: the position of some joints (elbow, wrist), and some new names of parts (dock, hock, fetlock, and forecannon).

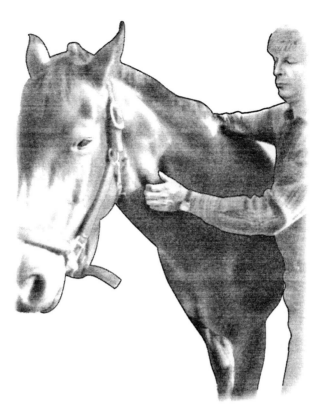

FIGURE 8–32. Massage therapist massaging a horse's neck muscles.

▪ LEARNING AND INTEGRATING APPROACHES

As you have discovered, many techniques overlap and might be labeled as integrated approaches. To avoid repetition in discussing the various methods, categories were chosen. Any excellent teacher or therapist is eclectic when putting together a specific massage for a specific client. So, to a certain extent, all massages are integrated.

Some of the therapies discussed here can be learned quickly and not all approaches can be certified by a larger body or institute. Students and clients should both be careful in choosing a therapy or a therapist. Ask to see diplomas and certification. Never believe anyone who tells you not to take your medications, not to see your physician, or that a therapy cures anything. Where there is little or no way to check a person's qualifications, fraud can be found.

Good therapists as well as good doctors and nurses have skills and understanding to minister to the human body. As you study this book and begin practicing, I ask you to learn from each client and to return again and again to the great books and the great teachers in this profession. The great healers I have known have excellent educations, human compassion, and a great touch. I wish you all the same.

▪ CASE STUDIES

1. The students of a massage school are going to a busy hospital today to give seated massage to its staff of doctors and nurses. These people are always stressed out and look forward to this weekly massage. Design a seated massage for them that is 15 to 20 minutes long.
2. Discuss a treatment plan for someone who has a contraindication to Swedish massage. Use one or more than one of the vibrational or energy techniques.
3. Choose a part of the body to concentrate on and learn the acupressure points for that body part. Do a Chinese or shiatsu treatment on that body part. Repeat again for another body part.
4. Ruth, 55, fell getting off a bus and dislocated her shoulder. She saw an osteopath, who repositioned the shoulder and suggested she get bodywork on it. She cannot get on a table and the shoulder is very sore. Use one or more of the muscle energy techniques to aid her limited range-of-motion and plan a treatment. When you can work on the shoulder, use an Oriental therapy to clear the whole meridian line affected. Plan a treatment for her.
5. Plan an integrated massage using a variety of strokes for your pet dog or cat.
6. Plan a massage using a variety of techniques with the primary goal of correcting a structural misalignment (a high, anteriorly rotated shoulder or a functionally short right leg). Focus on changing the structure throughout the massage and see if you can correct the misalignment.
7. Do a reflexology treatment on a friend or fellow student, using the chart provided in this chapter. First do the foot, then the hand, and finally, the ear.
8. Plan a complete treatment using a holding touch stroke and shaking and rocking of joints.
9. Do a lymphatic drainage massage on a fellow student or friend, concentrating on the arms or legs. Pump the proximal lymph nodes first with compression, and then work the proximal area very, very gently, repeating your strokes 5 to 7 times each. Finally, work the distal area of the limbs.
10. Devise a treatment plan using a variety of the modalities in this chapter. Tell why you are using them. Demonstrate the strokes to be used and ask for evaluation.

REVIEW QUESTIONS

1. Choose any five of the therapeutic approaches discussed in this chapter and describe them to another student.
2. Choose a modality in this chapter, and tell which strokes to use, when to use them, and why.
3. Describe how any of the modalities in this chapter might be incorporated into a regular massage.

4. Choose any of the modalities you did not know about before, and describe why you would or would not like to study it more.
5. How does a chin massage differ from a full body massage?
6. Define the vocabulary terms at the beginning of this chapter.

ASSESSMENT:
DESIGNING THE
MASSAGE TO FIT
THE CLIENT

Great ideas originate in the muscles.

Thomas Edison

LEARNING OBJECTIVES

After reading this chapter, students will be able to:

1. Construct a treatment plan from information gathered from health history forms, observations, questioning, and palpation (see Chapter 7 for coverage on each of these).
2. Use various techniques to assess clients.
3. Discuss case studies of clients and determine the therapeutic massage treatment appropriate to each.
4. Define the following vocabulary terms.

VOCABULARY TERMS

Assessment or	Objective assessment	SOAP notes
application	Plan, procedure,	Subjective assessment
HOPS	or progress	

▪ INTRODUCTION

Now is the time to put all the information you gathered in Chapters 7 and 8 together, perform the massage, and follow up with good notes. Once you have taken a health history, questioned the client about his or her responses (or lack of response), and ruled out any contraindications, you are ready to talk about a treatment plan for the client. Ask the client about troublesome areas, points of pain, onset of problems, and what he or she wants you to work on. You may need to know your client's job or profession, exercise activities, and any previous accidents and traumas. Begin to think about goals for this client. What can you reasonably accomplish today, or in the immediate future? What techniques will be best for this particular problem? Can this person lie on a massage table, or would a chair massage be better? Discuss your ideas for a treatment plan with the client. Palpate the areas discussed and see if you need to alter your plan. Get agreement from the client and write your plan down. If you need to change your plan because of things you find during the treatment, discuss it again with the client, get consent, and rewrite the plan after the treatment is over.

▪ ASSESSMENT

The assessment process (evaluation of the client) is complex and is often quickly dismissed by massage therapists in favor of hands-on techniques. However, if properly done, it can cut down on treatment time, be much more precise than treating everything and hoping to find something, and give the therapist a holistic view of problems. The following sections describe two of the best assessment tools, SOAP notes and the HOPS method. Together, these methods give you the client's thoughts and feelings about the problem as well as the therapist's, use palpation to confirm or deny any problems, and rely on special orthopedic tests, if needed, to settle any doubts about the region in question. Both the client's input and history and the therapist's intuition and physical assessment are critical to deciding on the treatment plan.

Good judgment and sound, educated decisions are based on a mastery of these evaluative skills.

SOAP Notes

Charting with **SOAP notes** is a way of organizing your observations and keeping original notes on your session with the client. SOAP stands for **Subjective assessment** (observation of behavior by client), **Objective assessment** (observation and behavior of client seen by therapist), **Assessment** or **application,** and **Plan, procedure,** or **progress** for present and future treatments. The SOAP note system was devised within the medical community and can be either very simple in its use or very tedious in its symbols. Appendix E gives the system organized for use in the massage profession. If you are going to work in a hospital or clinic, you will no doubt use the version already in place (Thompson, 1993).

While you are in school, use SOAP forms when you work on each other in class. Practicing now will greatly enhance your skills later when working on the public.

The skills needed to gather all this information, interpret it intuitively, and then apply a massage to suit the client's needs take time and practice to do well. It is a learning situation every time a therapist meets a new client. Someone once said at a massage school graduation that the students should go out and perform 1000 massages and then come back and ask their questions. I think many more times than that are needed to produce a master. Certainly, it is true in other disciplines.

HOPS Assessment Tool

The **HOPS** method (History, Observation, Palpation, and Special orthopedic tests) too, includes the history of the complaint, and observation and palpation of the client's overall condition as well as the area of complaint. This includes postural assessment. When needed, other tests such as special orthopedic tests will confirm or deny any suspicions the therapist might have about the area in question.

The history of the problem should be questioned thoroughly, with the client discussing the complaint. It may be the first time the client has told the entire story. Listen carefully for related problems, the nature of the pain, and the length of time since first incidence. Try to discover if the client has seen any other professional about the problem and if any change was made after that treatment. Also, seek to discover if daily activities benefit or aggravate the problem.

Under observation, do a postural assessment or body reading, which can begin when you first meet your client. (See Chapter 5.) Watch the client's gait and other movements as you listen to responses to your questioning.

During palpation of the areas involved, listen to your hands. They are your greatest tools. They will pick up information from the tissue itself and forward it to your brain for synergyzation with other information.

Special tests include both range-of-motion (ROM) testing for specific conditions and other orthopedic tests that isolate movements and muscles. Do both active and passive range-of-motion tests. For active ROM tests, note the following:

- Where and when the pain occurs.
- The client's reaction to the pain.
- Spasms or muscle splinting.
- Any restrictions.
- Client's willingness to move painful area.

For passive ROM, note end-feel restriction (bone to bone, hard or soft, tendon or muscle; a springy feel may indicate a loose body in joint; an empty feeling may be bursitis).

For resistive tests, the client may have:

- A muscle–tendon problem, if movement is strong and painful.
- A neuromuscular or joint injury, if movements are weak and painful.
- A neurological or severe tendon problem, if movement is weak and painless.
- No muscle–tendon problem, if movement is strong and painless.

▪ SPECIAL TESTS

Referrals

It may be necessary to refer your client to another professional for more testing procedures. These might include the following:

- *X-ray*. An x-ray is used to discover disorders of bones or joints; muscles do not show well on this test. An electromagnetic wave penetrates the tissues, and absorption of the wave displays the area on a photographic plate behind the tissues.
- *MRI*. Magnetic resonance imaging is painless and noninvasive. Nothing enters the skin. The patient enters the chamber while the machine produces images of the interior of the body.
- *CT*. Computerized tomography uses computer-enhanced images to show complicated structures or fractures deep within the body.
- *EMG*. Electromyography measures the contraction of a muscle as a result of electrical stimulation; it shows the neuromuscular components of soft tissues.
- *Myelogram*. This type of x-ray is used to detect spinal region problems. A dye or other medium is injected into the spinal column to reveal the presence of disc protrusions or lesions.
- *Isokinetic evaluation*. This method uses a computer-assisted strength resistance device to sense how much force a muscle is exerting during ROM testing.

Many tests have been developed for specific treatments, including piriformis or psoas test for sciatic nerve lesion and Phalen's test and Tinel's sign for carpal tunnel syndrome. See Chapter 11 for a more complete discussion of these and other tests and specific treatments.

Muscle Testing

Muscle testing has been used for many years by physical education professionals and some physicians to test the strength of muscles. By isolating a particular muscle and testing it, we can strengthen it, compare it to the same muscle bilaterally, or check its progressive improvement after injury.

Muscles can be tested with the client lying down or standing erect. First, isolate the muscle you wish to test. Position the body so that the ends of the muscle are close together. Press in a direction that requires the muscle you are testing to work to hold the body position (press against its pull). If the muscle gives way, or is shaky and baggy, it needs stimulation. (Thie, 1973). See Figure 9–1.

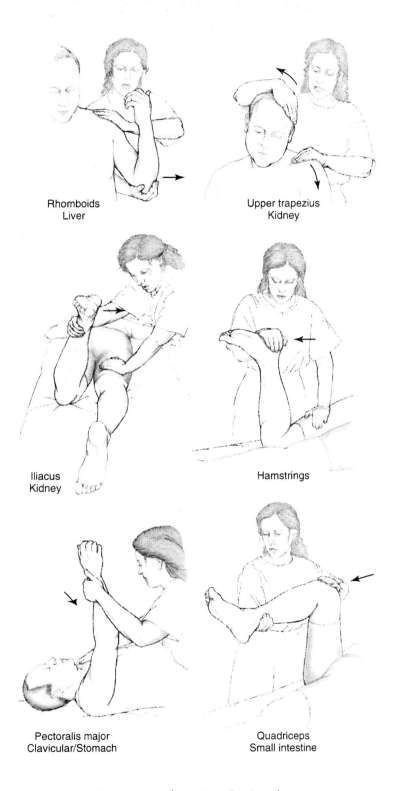

Rhomboids
Liver

Upper trapezius
Kidney

Iliacus
Kidney

Hamstrings

Pectoralis major
Clavicular/Stomach

Quadriceps
Small intestine

A

FIGURE 9–1. A. Muscle testing. *(Continued)*

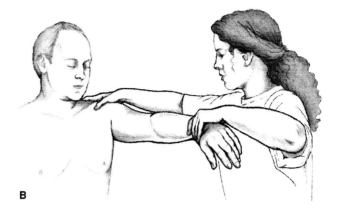

B

FIGURE 9–1 (cont.). B. Muscle testing on a client.

▪ ROUTINES

Sample routines are offered in Appendix E as a simple pattern for performing massage.

Before the Routine

Perform all the steps mentioned earlier in this chapter with the client before any massage, and position and drape the client on the table (see Chapter 6). Before any routine begins, practice the seven strokes enough to be familiar with them. In fact, it is a good idea to proceed through the strokes, doing a full body part or the entire body with each of the strokes in turn, so that you have enough experience with each of them to feel confident. It is also a good idea to walk through a routine first, doing no massage, until you are familiar with its steps. Then do the massage.

Reassessment After the Routine

After the massage has been completed, you and the client both want to know what changes have occurred. You can ask the client for movement of the area in question, ask what differences are sensed in that specific area, or retest the area using exactly the same test done in the same way as before the massage. Changes may occur after the client leaves the office, so asking the client to monitor any changes in the next 24 to 48 hours will help you design future treatments. This also keeps the client involved in the process, focusing on changes, not pain.

▪ QUICK ASSESSMENT TOOLS FOR CASE STUDIES

The following list of major assessment tools will help you prepare for case studies and for your massage practice:

1. Use the HOPS method to evaluate and assess soft tissue.
2. Note any limitation in range-of-motion of a joint. Test the uninvolved side first. Are daily activities impeded? Is there ease of movement?
3. Look for signs of inflammation (swelling, tenderness, heat, redness).
4. Listen for crepitus in joints, which suggests inflammation of joint or tendon sheaths.
5. Look for deformities using ROM, misalignment, dislocation.
6. Test muscular strength. Muscle weakness and atrophy may appear on one side only.
7. Look for symmetry of involvement on both sides of body (Fig. 9–2). Rheumatoid arthritis involves several joints. Misalignment itself can be the problem.

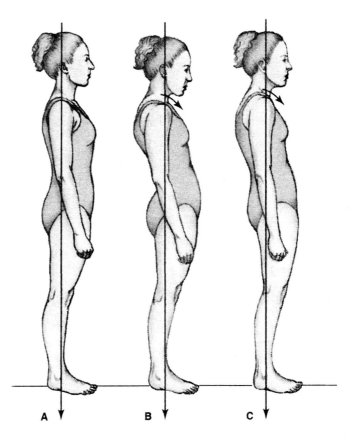

FIGURE 9–2. Balanced and imbalanced posture. **A.** Balanced alignment. **B, C.** Imbalances, which cause adaptations in connective tissue and in joints.

Some questions to ask the client follow, including questions on medical history and activities.

1. What is your primary complaint or problem? Listen carefully for pertinent details.
2. How did the pain occur? The nature of an accident is important, as is determining whether daily activity is affected or aggravated.
3. How long have you had this problem? You want to know if the problem is acute or chronic, and who else the client has seen about the problem.
4. How would you describe your pain? You want to know if it is sharp, burning, aching, electrical, and so forth.
5. Have you discovered any activities that make it better? Worse? You want to know the activities and movements that make it better or worse.
6. What is the client's occupation or job? Both work and weekend recreational activities may be related to the problem.
7. Have you ever had this problem before? Past injuries can give you ideas about this condition. Note how the past problem was resolved.

Practice asking these questions and others on health history forms to perfect your questioning skills. Then apply these assessment tools to the following case studies. Where no answers are given in the case study, such as in the ROM testing, create an answer that will help you to further your assessment skills, evaluation, and development of a treatment plan.

■ CASE STUDIES

1. Louise, age 45, is an infrequent regular for massage, coming for therapy every month or so. She works on computers in a busy hospital. Her upper back and neck muscles are tight, hard, and sore when worked. Louise could benefit from a full body massage to reduce stress and muscle tension, but she never gets it. She has had no accidents or trauma. Her health insurance does not cover massage.

   • Practice filling out a health history form for Louise or role-play an interview with her.
   • Devise a treatment plan for her and get consent if role playing.
   • Practice writing SOAP notes for this treatment session.
   • Practice doing the massage you would give her and ask for an evaluation afterwards.

2. Anne, a 55-year-old ectomorph (tall, skinny) who frequently injures her arms and legs, suffered a large contusion (a severe bruise due to a crushing, direct blow) on her upper arm. She was running to catch an elevator and it closed rapidly on her arm. As she was out of the country, she did nothing until she returned home. Then a physician assured her that no bones were broken and massage was suggested. There was an indentation in the

brachialis from the blow the muscle had taken. By this time, her arm was slightly discolored and the elbow was swollen. Her anterior arm was very sore to touch and both flexion and extension of the arm were affected.

- Practice palpating the affected muscles for heat, swelling, and tenderness by role-playing. Is there coolness due to ischemia?
- Do ROM movements to see restrictions in elbow extension and notice elastic end-feel and slight restriction in elbow flexion.
- Devise a treatment plan that will aid lymphatic drainage of the area, help restore muscle function, and reduce adhesions and deep scar tissue.
- Discuss treatment with the client and get consent.
- Do the massage and ask for evaluation.
- Practice writing SOAP notes for this session.
- Devise a treatment plan for long-term goals of eliminating adhesions, restoring ROM, and restoring strength to the arm.

3. John, a 40-year-old golf pro, had injured his right shoulder playing golf the day before. He receives massage only when he hurts. He felt a tear in a shoulder muscle when he was swinging. He did nothing, hoping the hurt would go away. He continued to play golf. Now, the next day, he is stiff and he wants you to "fix it."

- Take a health history by role-playing this case.
- Observe the client for pain or apprehension.
- Assess the injured site by palpation, looking for swelling, discoloration, tenderness, and alteration in the contours of the muscles; compare to the other arm.
- Test shoulder joint ROM. Mild strain would correspond to no pain throughout entire range-of-motion. With moderate strain, the joint is restricted and painful to move. With severe strain, ROM is impossible due to pain; refer to a physician.
- Prepare a treatment plan to increase lymphatic drainage and aid circulation to the arm.
- Maintain ROM by stretching muscles of the shoulder and use frictioning and stretches long-term to maintain healthy, mobile joint.
- Get informed consent, do massage, and get evaluated.
- Prepare SOAP notes for this session.

4. Josephine, a 34-year-old mother of two, comes to the clinic weekly for her massage. It is the highlight of her week. Today, she has a headache and sore neck muscles, probably caused by stress in her busy life. She would like to get rid of her headache and especially wants you to work on her neck.

- Discuss reasons for onset and severity of headache and sore neck muscles.
- Test ROM on neck.
- Devise a treatment plan for her massage.

- Perform the massage and ask for evaluation.
- Prepare SOAP notes for this session.

5. You have been asked to do an outreach experience for your school, using chair massage at the offices of a local, well-known corporation. You will perform several 15-minute massages on the employees (Fig. 9–3).

- Role-play or imagine several scenarios that the employees might present to you. (Overpowering, bossy manager who tells you what to do; overworked, underpaid employee who loves massage but cannot afford it; average worker who has never had massage and has no expectations.)
- Discuss client expectations and goals.
- Construct a treatment plan for each of the three roles given above.
- Perform the massage and ask for evaluation.
- Keep no records, just a sign-in sheet for the event.

6. Myra, 32, has the symptoms of TMJ (temporomandibular joint) syndrome. She has tension headaches, is undergoing a divorce, and is under

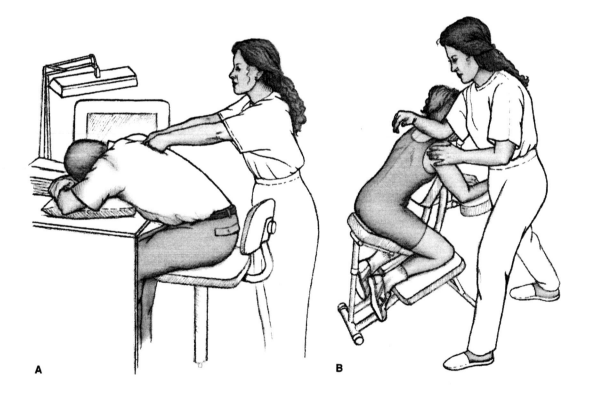

A   B

FIGURE 9–3. Seated massage **(A)** using ordinary chair and pillows and **(B)** in a gym. *(Continued)*

stress at her work. She has had no direct trauma to that area, but she often wakes up in the night grinding her teeth. When you palpate for trigger points on her jaw, you find several firing along the pterygoids and masseter.

- Determine how you should proceed if you have not received any special training in the treatment of TMJ.
- If you have had special training in TMJ treatments, list the questions you need to ask Myra and the observations needed for a postural assessment.
- What palpations need to be done for a thorough assessment? Do any testing needed.
- Devise a treatment plan for short- and long-term goals. Get informed consent.
- Do the massage and ask for evaluation.
- Create SOAP notes for this client.
- What remedial exercises may be needed, and what self-care can the client do as homework?

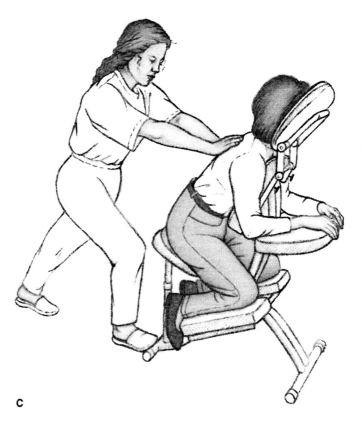

C

FIGURE 9–3 (cont.). Seated massage (**C**) in an office.

REVIEW QUESTIONS

1. Discuss the components that constitute a treatment plan.
2. Explain the meaning of SOAP notes.
3. Match the observation or interview information about a client to the correct portion of the SOAP notes (subjective = S, objective = O, application = A, plan = P).
   ___ a. Client looks ashen-faced and tired.
   ___ b. "My head hurts today."
   ___ c. Therapist will perform a full body massage.
   ___ d. Client's right shoulder is higher than the left.
   ___ e. Facial and scalp massage needed.
   ___ f. "My doctor told me I have sciatica."
   ___ g. Client can use hot packs on that muscle, no inflammation.
   ___ h. Swedish massage with trigger points around shoulder joints to reduce pain.
   ___ i. Next visit spend more time on hip rotation.
   ___ j. Therapist notices client's pain threshold is lowered today and pain is felt more often.
   ___ k. The alternative hot and cold packs seem to be helping stimulate the healing in that area.
   ___ l. "Nothing is helping me. I doubt you can do anything."
   ___m. Client is limping today.
   ___ n. Health history form states several accidents over the years, all involving whiplash.
   ___ o. Client's handshake is weak and he or she seems almost disinterested.
4. Define the vocabulary terms at the beginning of this chapter.
5. Describe some special assessment tests you can perform, and those that must be performed by another healthcare practitioner.

SELF-CARE
AND WELLNESS FOR
THERAPIST AND CLIENT

There is a secret person undamaged in every individual.

Paul Shepard

LEARNING OBJECTIVES

After reading this chapter, students will be able to:

1. Discuss the effects of stress and tension on the body, mind, emotions, and spirit.
2. Identify the signs of burnout as it applies to massage students and massage therapists.
3. Discuss and plan activities to reduce stress in their own lives and/or help their clients.
4. Discuss and demonstrate exercises and activities for themselves or their clients.
5. Define the following vocabulary terms.

VOCABULARY TERMS

Burnout	Gait	Tension
Diaphragmatic breathing	Stress	Yoga
Fight-or-flight response	Tai chi	

▪ STRESS AND TENSION

Much has been written about stress and its effect on the human body, mind, and soul. Certainly, everyone reading this book knows of its toll on him- or herself or someone else. Because stress is thought to be one of the main causes underlying disease, we will consider it again as we explore the therapist's world.

Tension and **stress** are the body's responses to change. Stress is present in almost every aspect of our lives just as change is everywhere. The body and mind attempt to meet fluctuations in the outside world and to maintain constancy or homeostasis in the inner world. Of course, some stress is needed in the body to maintain itself. Muscle contraction for posture and respiration keep us alive and upright. What we are discussing is the excess strain, which is perceived as beyond the body's or mind's adaptability. Such stress becomes "distress" or keeps us "under stress" and it is the response to such stress that we need to understand.

Hans Selye, the Canadian who first wrote in detail about stress (1978), identified three stages of stress. They are:

1. Alarm or **fight-or-flight response.**
2. Resistance response, in which the body continuously responds to the stress condition.
3. Exhaustion, which occurs if stage 2 continues without relief.

People respond differently to stress, and each of us has a different adaptive capacity. Risk factors such as diet, drugs, environment, age, lifestyle, gender, and genetic components moderate or intensify the body's response to stress.

As stress accumulates in the body and mind, it taxes our resources. The response can be as minor as sweating or evidenced in increased heart rate and respiration. It can include the fight-or-flight response, causing sweaty hands and a dry mouth. It can result in tension headaches, muscle contractions, and even stiff muscles. All of these are responses of the sympathetic nervous system. These responses can affect blood glucose levels, kidney function, and the immune system. The immune system suppresses its function, which allows bacteria and viruses to enter the body and take hold in times when a body is tired or inadequately nurtured. Chronic exposure to stress fatigues body systems so that their response to stress is altered and slowed. As a result, we can become more susceptible to disease, suffer from increased mental and emotional problems, and become more accident prone. Insomnia, overeating, smoking, panic attacks, alcohol and drug abuse, and more severe pathologies have all been related to the physiological changes produced by stress.

One of the primary aims of massage treatment is to decrease the sympathetic nervous system's response to stress, allowing a parasympathetic response of relaxation to occur. A safe, calm environment, relaxing music (if used), diffuse lighting, cool colors, secure draping, and a warm treatment all add to the relaxation of the client. During treatment, the therapist's voice should be calm and quiet. The conversation between therapist and client should be aimed at healing, as should working with the client's deep or **diaphragmatic breathing.** All these components of a successful massage also create a relaxing environment in which the body may restore itself.

▪ STUDENT AND MASSAGE THERAPIST BURNOUT

When a student enters massage school, he or she is usually unaware of the changes that are about to happen. In addition to the new discipline of study, interpersonal relationships with others in the class, and new demands on time outside of school, students are faced with personal growth. Massage is holistic in nature; it will bring to the forefront the issues and experiences that students need to confront in order to grow. Most people are not aware of this aspect of massage in the beginning of their schooling.

Because the body does store memory and events, these old experiences, traumas, and accidents are released from the body during massage. The student, having more massages in a week than many regular clients have in a month or a year, is faced time and again with past issues that need resolving and dissolving. This causes the massage student to face the facts and then let go. This process is not easy. It also can cause havoc at home, because many of our issues are family issues; the family may not wish to face these issues or to change, yet it is asked to deal with the changing massage student. Also, there is the pressure of time. Most massage students are in class less than one year. Tremendous changes are taking place every day of school in the body and mind, in the emotions and spirit. These changes are necessary, however, in order for the student to become a "healer."

A massage student can do several things to facilitate these changes that transform them from student to healer while they are in school (see Box 10–1).

Your life as a massage student will come to a successful conclusion, and suddenly you will find yourself in the hectic business world. For a short while, planning and setting up a new business will occupy your life. However, wherever you decide to work, you will be faced again with a new set of stress and tension factors. You want and perhaps need more clients. You do not have the time to yourself that you thought you would have. Certain clients are hard to deal with and you are worried about how to handle them. You need to continue your education to add to your knowledge, but time and money may be scarce. You work long and irregular hours. Some days you feel tired and perhaps your wrists, arms, or low back ache after working a full day. You are not exercising or eating as you know you should. You haven't had a massage yourself in weeks. Perhaps your mind and emotions are working overtime. You would like a vacation, but cannot think how you would manage it. The personal growth and/or personal fitness program you promised

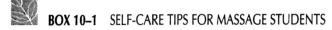

BOX 10–1   SELF-CARE TIPS FOR MASSAGE STUDENTS

- Stay positive; look to the end of the tunnel for light.
- Share learning experiences with family; don't shut them out.
- Discover your boundary lines in dealing with others (you will take this into your practice).
- Listen to people; don't tell them what to do.
- Watch your intake of caffeine, nicotine, and sugar; all affect learning abilities.
- Watch diet and exercise.
- Try to laugh a lot; it's good for your health and soul.
- Schedule regular massage treatments for yourself; exchange massage with another therapist, if necessary.
- Take care of your hands and arms.
- Find someone in the business with whom you can discuss your work.
- Take time for yourself, without guilt.
- Take up a new hobby, see a new film, visit a friend, read a new book.
- Continue your education.
- Take a vacation yearly, or more often if you can.
- Get plenty of rest.
- Work on your personal growth.
- Connect and ground yourself to the planet.
- Dream big in technicolor.

yourself while in school is no longer fitting into your schedule. In short, you are stressed out. This pattern of overwork, fatigue, poor diet and exercise, and lack of focus on wellness is **burnout.**

Many massage schools contact their graduates regularly after graduation. Their findings suggest that within a few years of becoming a massage therapist, many of these conditions have become a reality for a large portion of massage therapists.

Again, if we do not schedule wellness activities in our lives and make them a habit, stress will take over. Time for introspection, keeping up with massage literature, studying a new technique, eating correctly, and watching your posture and body mechanics leads you to become more relaxed, in better control of your life, and less likely to experience burnout. Burnout does not happen overnight. You will have warnings: fatigue, body aches from work, change in areas of your life, and workaholic tendencies. If these patterns begin to affect your ability to work and cope, it is time to change your lifestyle. Burnout is the effect of an undisciplined life. It will eventually make you ill and unable to work or to enjoy life as you once planned.

A plan to prevent burnout is necessary for our survival in this profession. Any plan we put into effect should consider the body, mind, emotions, and spirit since we are holistic in nature. Add ideas that suit your lifestyle to the self-care tips in the box. Notice that balance would be indicated if we would follow these tips. Balance in life outside will provide homeostasis inside. This is a sign of wellness.

▪ ACTIVITIES AND EXERCISES FOR SELF-CARE

Of course, this discussion of stress and stress reduction applies to your clients as well as to yourself. Once you are on a road to better health, you will be more helpful to your clients, and they will listen to you as someone who knows and does what you are suggesting to them. Both therapist and client may engage in any one or more of the following activities to help meet their goals of relaxation and stress reduction.

Yoga

Yoga is a form of mental control and exercise whose purpose is relaxation, breath control, and control over the body gained by performing a series of postures and body positions. When practiced regularly, yoga improves posture and muscle tone and relieves physiological and mental stress. This mental and physical discipline originated in India but has become popular in the Western world. To learn it correctly without doing physical harm to your body, you should study yoga with a qualified instructor (Fig. 10–1).

Tai Chi

Tai chi is a holistic system of exercise based on balancing the flow of energy in the body and the mind. The exercises are aimed at balancing the internal sources of imbalance, such as the emotional states of chronic anxiety, depression, and boredom;

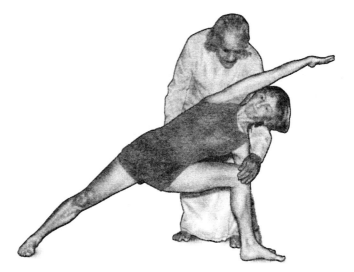

FIGURE 10–1. Yoga instructor and student. An instructor helps a student achieve the extended triangle posture in yoga (uttihita trikon asana). This posture tones leg muscles, removes stiffness in legs and hips, strengthens ankles, and develops the chest.

the physiological malfunctions such as organ weaknesses and congenital defects; and musculoskeletal misalignments such as congenital spinal problems and postural misalignments. It is important to maintain proper posture and alignment while doing exercises to create balance within the body. You can learn these exercises from a qualified instructor.

Deep Breathing Exercise

The action of diaphragmatic or deep breathing assures proper oxygen intake and release of carbon dioxide from the body. Breathing deeply is linked to autonomic nervous system patterns and is a total body experience, combining muscle contraction and relaxation. Many relaxation methods incorporate deep breathing as a crucial step in relaxation. There are several phases of both the inspiration and expiration steps of deep breathing (Fig. 10–2). For *inspiration*, the phases are as follows:

1. Quiet inspiration. Body at rest, the diaphragm and external intercostals are working.
2. Need for more oxygen. All muscles that pull ribs up are now working.
3. Forced inspiration. Body working hard, all previous muscles working along with shoulder girdle elevation muscles.

For *expiration,* the phases are as follows:

1. Quiet expiration. Passive. Muscles relax, thoracic wall recoils, gravity pulls rib cage down. No muscle action.
2. Freed expiration. Muscles pull down ribs and compress abdomen, forcing diaphragm upward.

In general, do deep breathing outdoors if you can. Breathe with the mouth closed; allow your nose to filter and warm the air.

Postural Correction Exercises

When assessing a client, use the outline suggested in Chapter 9. It is helpful to have a plumbline and a full-length mirror, but they are not necessary. Do a body reading and check the client's **gait** (manner of walking), standing and sitting position and plumbline view. Discuss your findings with the client afterwards and encourage body alignment as part of the relaxation process. Body parts work better when they are aligned; good function comes from good structure. Flexibility is an important part of building and maintaining well-being. The primary obstacles to flexibility are the musculature and fascia surrounding a joint. If the connective tissue surrounding a joint is encouraged to stretch on a regular basis, the normal range-of-motion of the joint will be maintained.

Day after day, the same movements at work or in exercise may cause overuse of the muscles and, over time, reduce flexibility. As a result, joints cannot maintain their normal range-of-motion. Here are 10 good reasons to stretch:

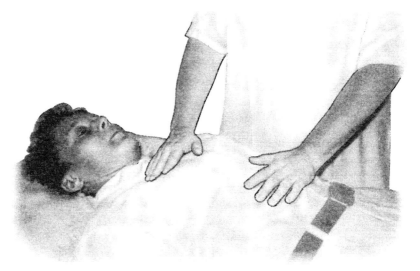

A. Inspiration

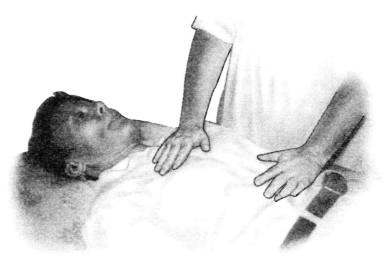

B. Expiration

FIGURE 10–2. Deep breathing exercises.

1. Decrease neuromuscular tension and reduces stress.
2. Improve the capacity for activity; stretched muscles require less energy for movement.
3. Relieve muscle soreness.
4. Increase and maintains a complete range-of-motion (ROM) of the joint.
5. Relieve muscle–joint stiffness associated with aging.

6. Stretch the fascia that binds the connective tissue together.
7. Increase tissue temperature in warm-up and warm-down processes.
8. Increase athletic potential.
9. Reduce tightness that may contribute to pain, spasm, or cramping.
10. Aid recovery during rehabilitation.

General Principles About Stretching

Efficient stretching begins by identifying and isolating a specific muscle or muscle group. Next, the contraction of either the agonist or antagonist muscle should be intensified. At this point, these two muscles alternate in relaxing and lengthening around the joint involved.

Breathing regularly during muscle exertion decreases the fatigue associated with the waste product lactic acid, which is formed as the muscle burns glucose for fuel. Inhale as the body returns to the starting position, exhale during the working phase of stretching.

A warm-up period and a warm-down period are important to prevent injury of the musculotendinosis unit, reduce recovery time, and allow the heart rate to return to normal slowly after the stretching period. A warm-up could include walking, gentle running, or use of a stationary bicycle. Warm-downs can reduce cramping and stiffness and promote relaxation following an activity.

Ballistic stretching or bouncing motion is not recommended. It can cause muscle tears, overtensed muscles, and "stretch reflex," which causes rapid contraction within the muscle due to the spindle cells receiving a message to prematurely stretch. This can cause spasms and pain.

Range-of-motion will be increased if the stretching exceeds the existing ROM. Always move beyond the point of slight irritation. Hold for 1 to 2 seconds, release, return to starting position, and repeat several more times. Thus, the reversal contraction of the tissue triggered by the stretch relax will be bypassed, and you will likely avoid soreness from overstretching and not encounter tissue tearing and the formation of scar tissue.

Take your time and gradually increase your flexibility. Your positive mental attitude and ability to relax will go a long way to help you achieve added flexibility.

Postural exercises such as stretching the spine and back, abdominal curls, leg swings, bicycling while on the back, lumbar twist, and knee to chest extensions can all be done to enhance posture. The yoga positions of the cobra, bow pose, lotus, and tailor-sitting all encourage good posture.

Self-Stretching Exercises

Self-stretching exercises are those the therapist or client can do on his or her own. They may rely on other parts of the body, gravity, or objects about the house. Examples follow; repeat each exercise 8 to 10 times.

1. To stretch muscles of the low back and hips, lie face up on the floor. With one arm, grasp the opposite knee and pull to chest. Repeat with the other arm and leg (Fig. 10–3).

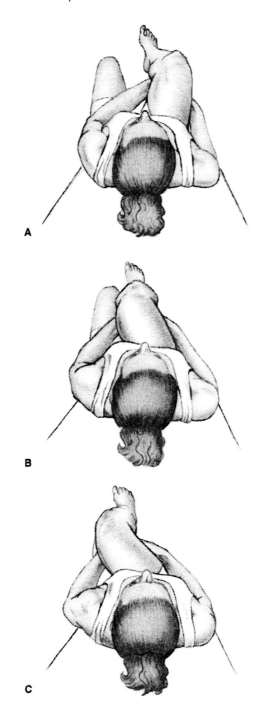

FIGURE 10–3. Low back and hips stretch. **A.** Single knee straight to chest. **B.** Single knee to center chest. **C.** Single knee to opposite shoulder.

Bend both knees and make a circular motion with your knees. Do tiny circles first and then make them larger. Reverse the direction (Fig. 10–4).

In a sitting position, left leg straight, bend the right leg and cross it over the outside of the left leg (Fig. 10–5). Place right hand upon lower right leg. Take a breath and slowly turn toward the left side of the body. Inhale and return to the beginning position. Turn again to the left and stretch a little farther, exhaling as you turn. Your aim is to be able to look behind you, over your left shoulder. Repeat on the other side.

2. To stretch the hamstrings, stand and place one leg forward and held straight on a low hassock or stool. Bring the chest towards the knee and keep the back straight. Repeat 10 times (Fig. 10–6A).

Lie on your back, with right leg resting on a bolster or pillow, left leg bent. Place a rope under the right foot. Hold both ends of the rope in your hands. Slowly inhale as you tighten the abdominal muscles and raise the leg toward a 90-degree position. Do not use force. Repeat on other side. Repeat two sets of 10 times each (Fig. 10–6B).

3. To stretch the piriformis, lie on your back on a massage table, bolster or pillow under the knees. Rotate left leg inward, toes turned towards the medial line of the body. Place a rope under the foot, holding the ends of the rope in

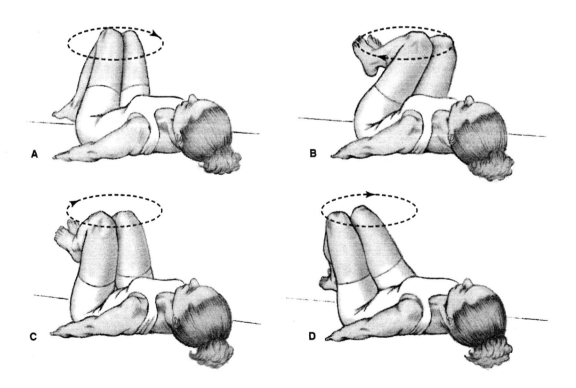

FIGURE 10–4. Circles. Bend both knees and make a circular motion with your knees.

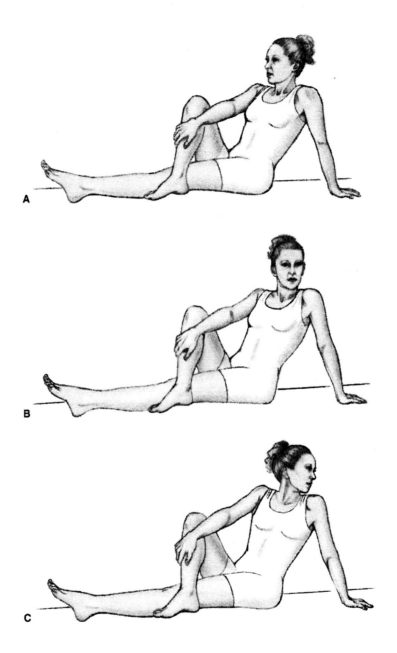

FIGURE 10–5. Hip rotator stretch.

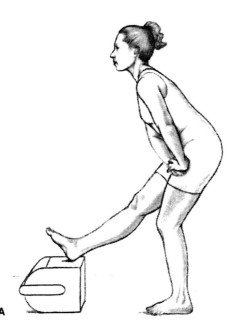

FIGURE 10–6. A. Hamstring stretches. *(Continued)*

the left hand. Raise the leg to 90 degrees. Lower leg slowly towards the table while whole leg is over the midline of the body. Keep shoulders and pelvis on the table. Keep the leg rotated, do not turn the waist. When the leg is completely lowered, it will be at a 90-degree angle to the straight leg, lying across it, leg pointing left. Repeat 10 times (Fig. 10–7).

To stretch the psoas, lie on your back on a massage table with your head in the center of the table and pelvis near the right side edge. Flex both knees. Repeat 10 times. Bring left knee to left side of the chest. Place both hands under the left foot to hold this position. Slowly move the right leg down toward the table. The upper right leg should be able to rest on the table. Do not allow the pelvis to tilt or the back to arch (Fig. 10–8).

4. To stretch the shoulder, stand straight. One hand crosses the body and grasps the opposite shoulder. Push the shoulder back and increase the stretch by using the free hand to push on the opposite elbow. Repeat 8 to 10 times (Fig. 10–9A, C).

Sit on a massage table or the floor. Flex legs, cross ankles, and wrap arms around the knees. Take a deep breath, tuck chin, and roll head downwards one vertebra at a time. Exhale and move slowly. Inhale as you move the head up, expand the chest, and look above eye level. Tuck the chin, exhale, and move downward towards chest. Repeat while turning towards the right knee. Repeat until the head can rest on the right knee. Repeat turning to left side and left knee. Repeat several times (Fig. 10–9B).

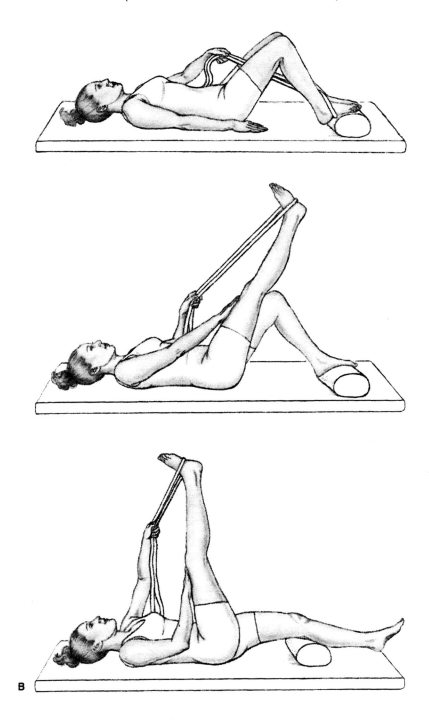

FIGURE 10–6 (cont.). B. Using a rope to stretch the hamstrings.

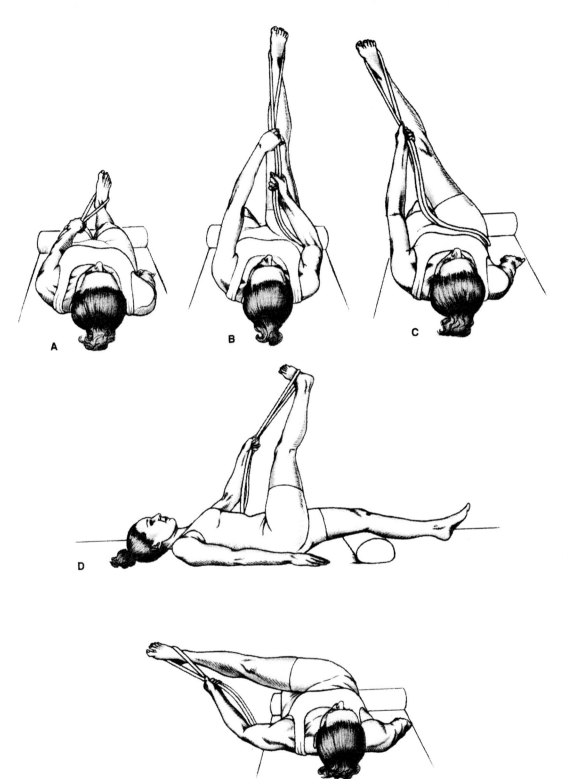

FIGURE 10–7. Piriformis stretch.

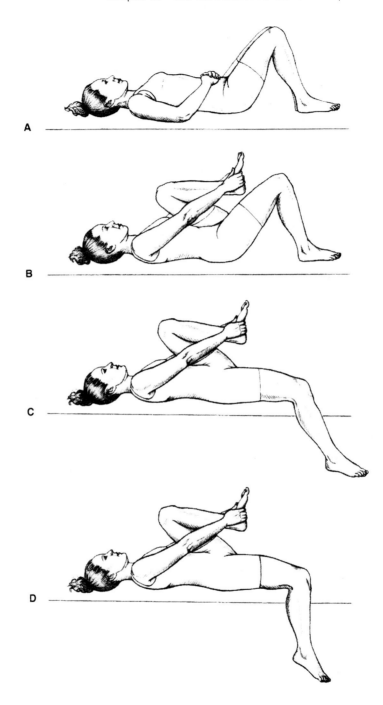

FIGURE 10–8. Psoas stretch.

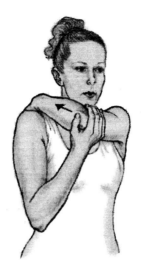

FIGURE 10–9. Shoulder stretches. *(Continued)*

To stretch the anterior shoulder, stand straight and thrust both arms and hands behind you. Grab your hands together and push backwards and upwards at the same time. Repeat 8 to 10 times (Fig. 10–9C).

5. To stretch the back, stand, arms at your sides. Take a deep breath as you raise your head upward and look above eye level. Exhale as the upper body leans slowly backward. The low back arches slightly as the neck and chest are stretched. Inhale and return to the erect position. Repeat 8 to 10 times (Fig. 10–10).

Lie on your stomach with arms at sides of body. Inhale normally. Exhale and slowly raise the head and look above eye level. Inhale as you return the head to the table. With each breath, raise the head a little higher. Repeat 8 to 10 times (Fig. 10–11).

Lie on your stomach with arms bent shoulder high, chin resting on table. Exhale as you raise the head. Look above eye level. Continue exhaling as the arms push off and the head and upper body rise up higher. Repeat 8 to 10 times (Fig. 10–12).

Care of Hands and Arms

Among the most important areas of the body that therapists need to exercise and strengthen are their hands and arms. After all, these are most important in delivering a massage to another person. Often, students and new therapists do not pay enough attention to these limbs and they become tension-ridden, sore, achy, hard, and eventually so painful that giving massages becomes impossible. Nerve damage or carpal tunnel syndrome may result.

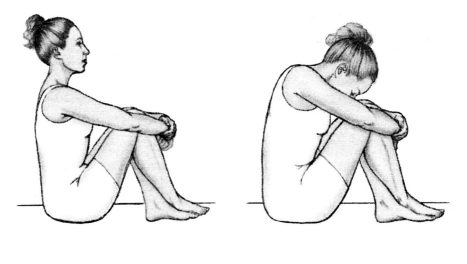

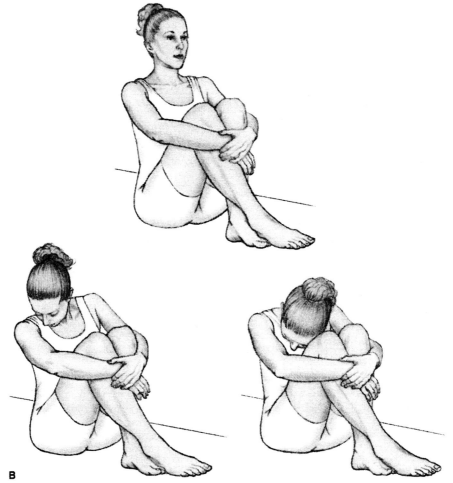

B

FIGURE 10–9 (cont.). Shoulder stretches.

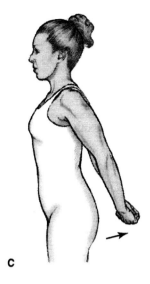

C

FIGURE 10–9 (cont.). Shoulder stretches.

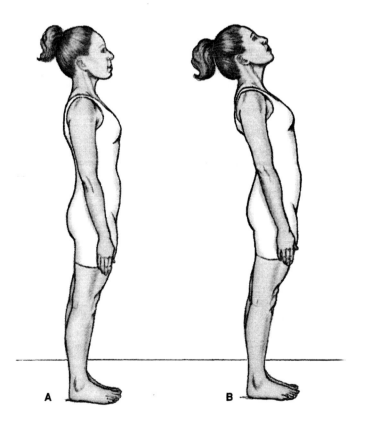

A   B

FIGURE 10–10. The back arch standing.

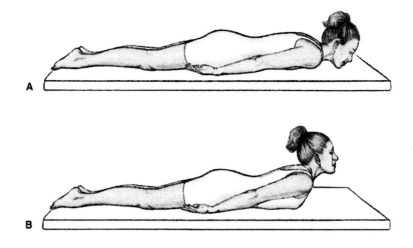

FIGURE 10–11. The back arch lying down.

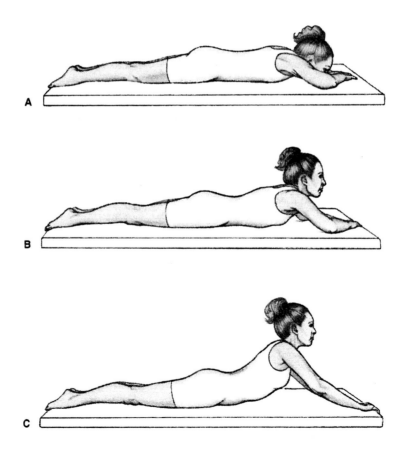

FIGURE 10–12. Variant of lying back arch.

There are suggested treatments and exercises that you can do as a therapist to protect and aid your hands and arms to prevent injury. As soon as you start massage school, begin to exercise your hands to develop their strength, flexibility, and control.

- Exercise to strengthen your arms, shoulders, and hands. Clasp your hands behind your back at the waistline or just below the waistline and pull your arms outward and upwards, holding for 10 seconds. Pull arms downward for 10 seconds. (This exercise can also be given to clients for drawing back their shoulders to a better position.) See Figure 10–13.
- Exercise to shake off energy, relax, and warm the hands. Hold your hands chest high and shake them vigorously for 10 seconds (Fig. 10–14).
- Play a piano or type on a flat surface to improve hand control and coordination. Make sure you tap with each finger several times (Fig. 10–15A).
- Hold your hands in the air and rotate the wrists in both directions to make a circle. Repeat 10 times each way. This exercise strengthens and limbers the wrists (Fig. 10–15B).

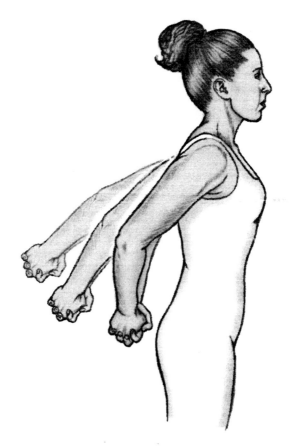

FIGURE 10–13. Exercise to strengthen arms, shoulders, and hands.

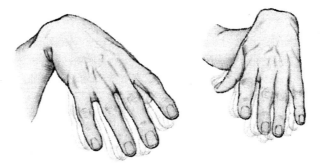

FIGURE 10–14. Exercise to shake off energy, relax, and warm the hands.

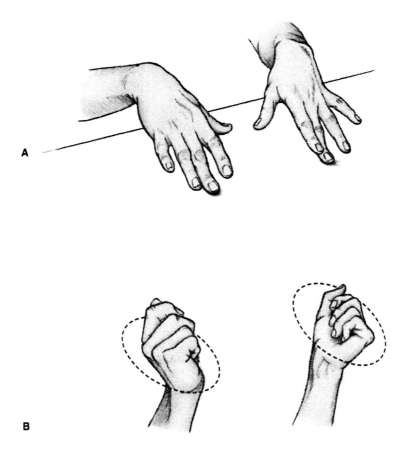

FIGURE 10–15. A. Playing a piano or typing on a flat surface. **B.** Making circles.

- With one hand pressing the other, hold your palms pressed together, applying alternate force each against the other. Repeat 10 times. This exercise helps the wrists to become strong and supple (Fig. 10–16A).
- Press the fist of one hand into the other hand while resisting. Repeat 10 times. This exercise strengthens the entire arm and hand (Fig. 10–16B).

Other suggestions for strengthening and detoxifying the hands and arms are given in Box 10–2.

Relaxation, Meditation, and Visualization Tapes

The marketplace today is flooded with tapes for every conceivable condition that needs our attention. Many of them are excellent; some are not. Performers such as

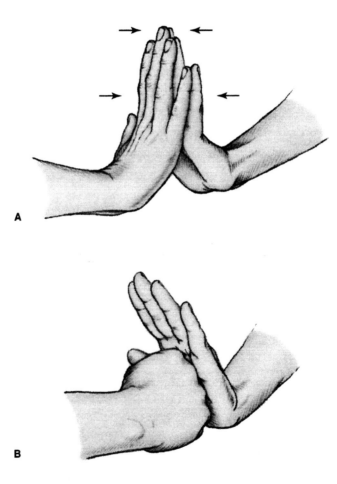

FIGURE 10–16. Hand positions. **A.** One hand pressing the other. **B.** One hand pressing a fist into the other hand.

BOX 10-2   HAND CARE

- Massage each finger, hand, and arm every day to remove stress and tension.
- Dip the hand into and/or paint the arm with hot wax paraffin as in a paraffin bath each day. This encourages healing of the area.
- Fill a balloon with sand. (Do not blow up the balloon first.) Tie the end of the balloon and use it as a ball to squeeze.
- When arms ache, soak them in hot water and Epsom salts for 10 to 15 minutes. Use one pound of Epsom salts in a basin of hot water.
- Secure a soft putty ball from a sports store. (They come in various strengths.) Squeeze as you watch television. Hold the ball with the thumb and first finger and squeeze and roll ball between other fingers. Repeat with other hand. After a month or so, get a harder ball (Fig. 10–17).
- Obtain a pair of Chinese medicine musical balls. Place them in your palms and rotate them in your hands, twirling them around all fingers. The music they produce is added therapy for your ears (Fig. 10–18).
- Obtain a Gyroflex yoyo-like ball that activates and moves your hands and arms in all directions. Use on both hands to improve circulation and build strength (Fig. 10–19).

Stephen Halpern, Yanni, and others put out excellent tapes for the massage therapist to use in his or her practice. You can obtain meditation tapes and visualization tapes that aid relaxation and guide you in visualization techniques. There are even whole series of nature tapes that transport you to a variety of regional environments. These tapes can be found in New Age bookstores, music outlets, and some larger bookstores.

Please be sure to get informed consent from clients before using a subliminal tape that might aid them. It would be unethical to use one without their knowledge. Always ask clients what they wish in the music for their session; tastes vary a great deal among people.

Journaling

Another technique that aids relaxation is the act of writing each day in a journal. This allows us to process what is happening to us and our response to it while it is fresh in the mind. Often, the art of telling an incident or writing it down frees it from the body. At any rate, we can then explore it and its effect on us without storing it in the body's memory. We can see the accumulation day by day of things that affect us. Then we can do something about them.

Touch for Health

Yet another technique uses the activities associated with touch for health, a modality associated with massage that uses applied kinesiology. This self-help system of

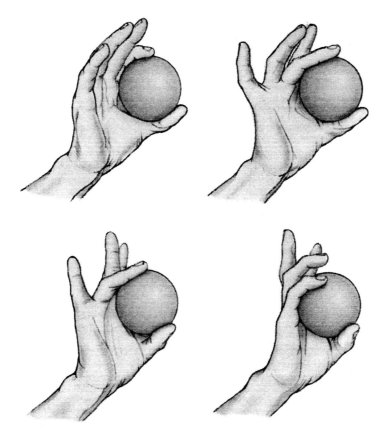

FIGURE 10–17. Squeezing a rubber or foam ball.

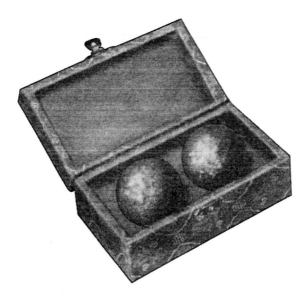

FIGURE 10–18. Chinese musical balls.

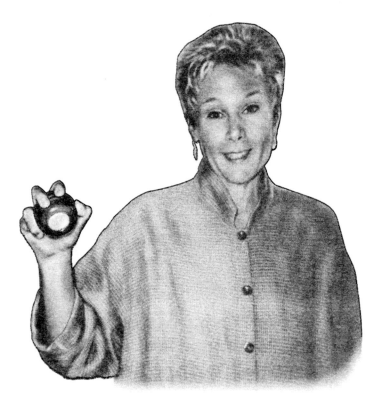

FIGURE 10–19. Gyroflex ball. Self-activated yoyo-like ball that moves your hands and arms in all directions.

muscle testing and the holding of acupressure points has the aim of restoring balance to the energy system of the body (Thie, 1973).

REVIEW QUESTIONS

1. Discuss the three stages of stress in the body.
2. Discuss the effects of stress and tension on the body, mind, emotions, and spirit.
3. Identify the signs of burnout as a massage student and as a massage therapist.
4. Discuss several activities to reduce stress.
5. Describe posture-correcting and self-stretching exercises.
6. Define the vocabulary terms at the beginning of this chapter.

THERAPEUTIC MASSAGE: THE APPLICATION OF KNOWLEDGE TO CLIENT NEEDS

The body never lies.

Martha Graham

LEARNING OBJECTIVES

After reading this chapter, students will be able to:

1. Identify and discuss the general indicators of inflammation and pain and understand their role in certain pathologies.
2. Discuss the three steps of inflammation and the three steps of pain.
3. Discuss the various forms of hydrotherapy and how they should be used.
4. Devise massage treatments for local concerns such as edema, scars, strains, sprains, and whiplash.
5. Adapt massage components to apply them to specific treatments.
6. Identify the massage needs of special populations, and be able to devise massages for the pregnant mother, infant, athlete, elderly, and chronically and terminally ill.
7. Define the following vocabulary terms.

VOCABULARY TERMS

Adhesion	Hydrotherapy	Systemic inflammation
Affusion	Paresthesia	Thalassotherapy
Cryotherapy	Phantom pain	

▪ GENERAL PATHOLOGIES AND MASSAGE TREATMENTS

Before we begin a discussion of massage treatments for pathologies, we'll review and expand on the discussion of pain and inflammation in Chapter 3.

Inflammation

Inflammation is a local response to tissue injury. This response is the body's method of minimizing tissue injury and maintaining homeostasis. The cause of tissue damage may be internal or external. Trauma such as a blow to a body part, infection, surgery, ischemic damage, chemical damage, or radiation damage may occur, but the response will be the same. The three stages of inflammation are as follows.

Acute Stage. In the first several days of injury (days 1 to 4), the area becomes red and warm to the touch, swelling occurs, and there may be pain, muscle spasm, and reduced range-of-motion. The causes of these changes are immediate vasoconstriction, then vasodilation; capillary beds leak fluid to the interstitium (exudate formation) and toxins are diluted. This limits the spread of bacteria. Clot formation follows, as does phagocytosis of the injurious agent. The bacteria and damaged cells are filtered in the lymph nodes and destroyed by white blood cells. Often, lymph nodes enlarge due to the infectious material.

If tissue damage is severe, the inflammation response is excessive, or the causal agent is not eliminated, collagen formation will increase and adhesions of tissue will occur. **Adhesions** are the abnormal connections of tissue layers.

Subacute Stage. In the second phase of the inflammatory process (days 4 to 14), the formation of loose connective tissue begins. Fibroblasts and collagen form a ground substance matrix. Capillary beds expand into the injured site to provide a blood supply. Adhesions may begin. The pain and swelling will go down, but muscle weakness and decreased range-of-motion (ROM) may occur due to adhesions.

Chronic Stage. In the third stage of inflammation (days 14 to 21), the connective tissue matures and begins to constrict the scar tissue. The collagen aligns itself in the direction of stress. Decreased function because of restriction of movement and adhesion formation may result. Muscle weakness and pain may remain. This chronic stage can last years. Tendonitis may recur, which can increase the risk of future damage, rescarring, and deformity.

Treatment Concerns of Inflammation. The treatment concerns in an inflammatory condition in the acute stage would be to limit the effects of the inflammation. Rest, ice, compression, and elevation (RICE) would be applied to the injured part. The focus of any treatment would be to the rest of the body that is not injured, such as relaxing the person and maintaining ROM of unaffected joints. For edema and pain, local use of cold hydrotherapy is suggested. Proximal work is indicated to the injured site and distal techniques are used carefully.

In the subacute stage of inflammation, as the inflammation subsides, a minimum of pressure and working within the pain tolerance of the client are primary. Gentle frictions and stretching to realign connective tissue may be used. Take care not to reinjure the area, as the new tissue is very fragile. Ice may be used after massage to limit inflammation.

In the chronic stage of inflammation, treatment should focus on the function of the site and on compensating structures. Hot hydrotherapy can be used; remedial exercise and strokes are more vigorous. Any adhesions formed need to be broken down and muscle spasms and trigger points should be addressed. Assessment of the client's ability to perform daily tasks is important at this stage, as is any postural reeducation that is necessary.

When inflammation becomes **systemic inflammation,** changes affecting the whole body occur and the condition is known as inflammatory disease. Antihistamines can suppress inflammation by blocking the actions of histamine. Therapeutic massage seems to be beneficial, as it appears to help:

1. Release the body's own anti-inflammatory agents.
2. Speed up the process by increasing the inflammatory process.
3. Dilute and remove the irritant by increasing lymphatic drainage.

Pain

Pain is complex, subjective, poorly defined, and difficult to understand (Box 11–1). It is important that when a client complains of pain, the therapist must believe it exists. Pain is one of the main reason the client needs help. For the therapist, pain helps to locate the cause of disease.

The definition of pain states that it is unpleasant and is caused by noxious stimulation of the sensory nerve endings. Pain receptors, nociceptors, are the branch endings of dendrites of sensory neurons. Excessive stimulation causes pain to be felt. Injured tissue may release prostaglandins, making nociceptors more sensitive. Aspirin and other anti-inflammatory drugs inhibit their release and thus relieve pain. The body has many reactions to pain. Pain proceeds from the affected area to the spinal cord, and travels to the thalamus and cerebral cortex, where it is modulated.

Acute pain is usually a symptom of a disease. Called bright or pricking pain, it acts as a warning, comes on suddenly, is easily located, and is temporary. Often, it goes away by itself.

Chronic pain is a problem for a good portion of society. Called aching or burning pain, it is hard to locate, changes places and intensity over time, and is hard to

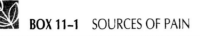

BOX 11-1   SOURCES OF PAIN

- Cutaneous pain is superficial, local, bright, burning, sharp, from tissue damage.
- From deeper somatic structures, pain is more diffuse and refers to other parts of the body.
- Visceral pain is diffuse and is caused by abnormal contraction or ischemia of the gastrointestinal tract.
- Functional or psychogenic pain arises from the emotions or psyche but is felt as if it arose from organic causes.

---

diagnose. Pain felt over 6 months' time is considered chronic. Even when treatment is given, chronic pain can become intractable pain.

Intractable pain is very difficult to remove. Known as deep pain, it often exists when there is no disease process and when treatment is given. Massage aids this type of pain for a short time only. Be prepared to have it travel around the body from place to place. It takes a long time to eliminate.

Phantom pain is sometimes felt by clients who have had an amputation of a limb. The pain in the leg, for instance, feels as if the limb was still present. In fact, some people believe that the blueprint of the body still exists and that the limb can still be felt in the client's aura. Others believe the remaining sensory nerves have been further stimulated by the amputation and the trauma, thus causing the pain. In any case, massage is indicated.

Pain can be localized and confined to the origin site. Pain can be projected to nearby the original site as a result of proximal nerve compression. Pain can radiate and become diffused around the original site. Pain can be referred to a distant area away from the original site (Fig. 11–1).

There are two responses to pain—physical and psychological. The physical response to pain includes increased blood pressure, sweating, and a shift of the blood flow from the brain and stomach to the muscles in preparation for "fight-or-flight." The psychological response to pain includes tension, stress, fear, and anxiety. It differs from person to person depending on the previous experience of pain. Only the client perceiving the pain can identify its intensity.

Fortunately, massage can help to alleviate pain at slight or moderate levels. If a client is experiencing extreme pain, a physician referral is in order. Sometimes massage can help reduce the pain enough to allow reduction in medications or some side effects of the medications.

Endorphins and enkephalins are produced by the body to moderate pain perception. The former are found in the limbic system and other brain stem structures, while the latter are found in the midbrain, hypothalamus, and dorsal horn of the spinal cord. Norepinephrine is produced by the sympathetic nervous system and can also block pain.

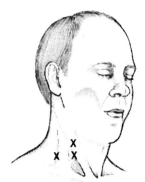

A. Active trigger points in the platysma refer a strange prickling pain to the mandible area and sometimes to the chest.

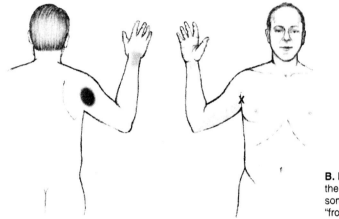

B. Pain associated with the subscapularis muscle sometimes resembles a "frozen shoulder."

FIGURE 11–1. Referred pain diagrams emanating from nearby trigger points. *(Continued)*

Massage can also release these morphine-like chemicals in the brain, so that pain is modified or eliminated. Massaging an area in pain increases the circulation of that area so that both increased blood flow and increased lymphatic draining are helping to restore the area. Moist heat acts similarly to massage. Remaining trigger points can be treated with ischemic compression and muscle stripping, followed by passive stretching. This restores muscle length and joint ROM.

The cycle of dysfunction–pain–voluntary splinting–restricted movement–more dysfunction can become a vicious cycle and sometimes continues long after the original injury has healed (see Chapter 3).

Again, it needs to be emphasized that anyone with an unexplained pain pattern should be referred to a physician. Pain has physical, psychological, social, and financial components. A massage therapist's role is to offer a supportive and non-judgmental environment in which both the therapist and the client seek to alleviate pain.

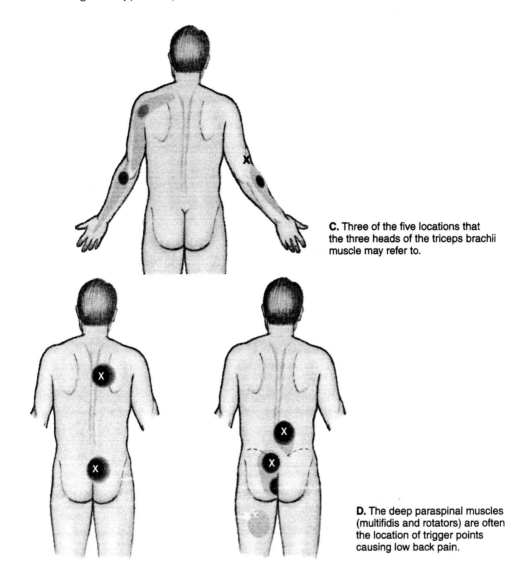

C. Three of the five locations that the three heads of the triceps brachii muscle may refer to.

D. The deep paraspinal muscles (multifidis and rotators) are often the location of trigger points causing low back pain.

FIGURE 11–1 (cont.).

▪ USE OF HYDROTHERAPY AND SPA TREATMENTS

Hydrotherapy is a form of therapy that uses water in any of its forms either internally or externally. It combines very well with massage, as it aids in balancing the body, removing toxins, and softening tissues. Like massage, it can stimulate the body or relax it, depending on its use. It can be used locally, for example, on constricted muscles to soften them, encourage circulation and lymphatic drainage, and prepare the muscles for massage. It can also be used over the whole body, as in providing contrasting hot and cold baths or showers to stimulate overall healing, increasing circulation, increasing relaxation, and reducing and then later increasing nervous tension. Cells are stimulated to function normally. Only therapists who have been trained thoroughly in the techniques of hydrotherapy should use it with their clients.

Bathing and water techniques have been used in therapy as long as humans have been near water. From classical Greece onward, written accounts document such bathing techniques used for therapeutics. Today, spas are enjoyed by people on every continent and are available to millions, no matter where they may live. If there is no spa near you, you can create one by your use of hydrotherapy in your practice.

There are a few good books on the subject. Among them are *Manual of Hydrotherapy and Massage* (Moor et al., 1964) and a book combining hydrotherapy and heliotherapy, *Natural Healing With Water, Herbs and Sunlight* (O'Rourke, 1995). Get training in the subject before you use it in your practice.

Types of Hydrotherapy

- *Local cold application* (**cryotherapy**). Cold compresses, ice lollipop, ice bag, vasocoolant such as fluoromethane sprays (Fig. 11–2).
- *Local heat application.* Moist, hot compresses; thermaphores; wax baths; hydrocollator pads; hot water bottle.
- *Hot and cold frictions.* Use of loofah, face cloth, mitten using hot or cold water to rub the body. Herbals are often added to the water. A tonic effect is produced.
- *Compresses and packs.* To cover a wider area, use cotton, flannel, or gauze soaked in herbal or medicated water. A hydrocollator or moist heat packs are often used (Fig. 11–3).
- *Sprays* (**affusions**) or *showers.* One or several streams of water are aimed at the body at the same time and can be alternated.
- *Baths.* Any part of the body or the whole body may be immersed in any temperature water or steam (foot bath, sitz bath, full bath, steam bath).
- *Steam.* A steam room, vaporizer, steam inhalation (a towel draped over the client's head and a bowl filled with very hot water, or steam cabinet (Russian bath) (10 to 15 minutes) is used to produce profuse perspiration, relaxation, and improved metabolism (Fig. 11–4 and Box 11–2). Steam applications can help to add moisture to the air and cleanse the system of impurities.
- *Sauna.* A heated room with dry heat. Very intense. Dehydrates the body, but removes toxins. Drink water afterwards and take a tepid shower.
- *Swedish shampooing.* A cleansing bath given on a massage table, using brush or bath mitt or loofah, soap, and water.
- *Jacuzzi, whirlpool, or hot tubs.* Large tubs with jets and/or agitators of the water under pressure that can be aimed underwater at specific body parts. Causes relaxation.
- *Salt glow.* Sea salt is rubbed into the skin and then rinsed off.
- *Body wraps.* Sheets or towels are dipped in herbal water, wrung out, and tightly wrapped around the body.

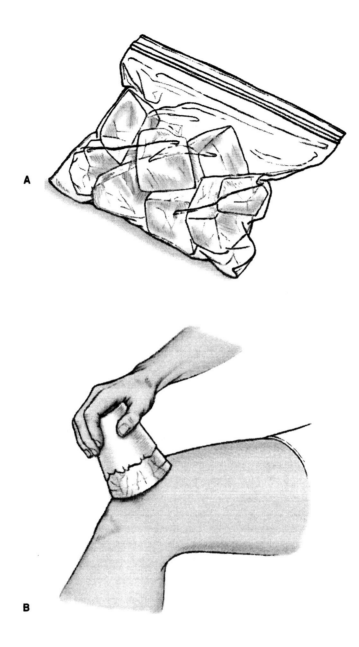

FIGURE 11–2. Cryotherapy. **A.** Inexpensive ice pack. Sealed plastic bag with ice cubes. For a quick alternative, use a package of frozen vegetables from the freezer. **B.** Water frozen in a styrofoam cup is applied as ice massage.

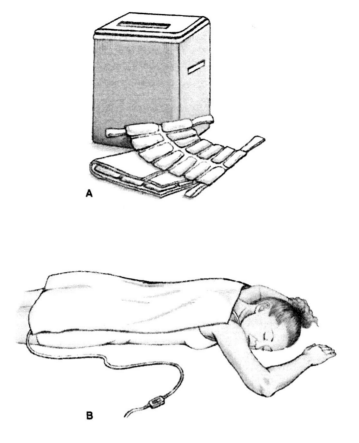

FIGURE 11–3. Moist heat. **A.** Moist heat packs heated in a hydrocollator filled with heated water and then applied to the body. The silica gel inside the packs maintains the heat. Normally, they are covered with a terrycloth cover or towel before use. **B.** Electric moist heat or fomentation pad.

Contraindications for Hydrotherapy

Persons with diabetes, kidney infection, cardiac impairment, lung disease, high or low blood pressure, or infectious skin conditions should not receive hydrotherapy. Check with a physician if you are not sure about a specific client.

Effects of Cold Water

The short-term effects of cold water on the body include improved circulation, stimulation of the nerves, and improvement in the cell activity (Box 11–3). The long-term effects of cold have a depressing effect on the body and should not be used unless the client is under supervision.

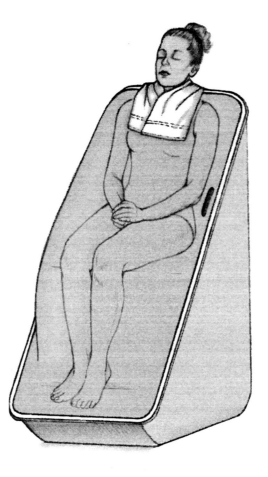

FIGURE 11–4. Russian bath or steam cabinet bath.

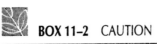 **BOX 11–2** CAUTION

Do not leave a person in a steam cabinet without supervision. Lots of water should be consumed to offset loss of fluids from the body. Remove the client from the cabinet if headaches or throbbing in the head occurs. Place cold compresses on the forehead and/or the back of the neck.

BOX 11-3   IMMEDIATE EFFECTS OF CRYOTHERAPY

- Chills the skin, stimulates it.
- Contracts surface blood vessels and drives blood to the interior of the body; increases circulation.
- Reduces leukocyte migration; lymph activity slowed.
- Reduces nerve sensitivity, reduces pain, has an analgesic effect.
- Slows the functional activity of cells; tissue stiffens, muscle tone increases.
- Reduces inflammation.
- Slows metabolism.

Use of Cold Water or Ice (Cryotherapy)

For Injuries. Use an ice bag or pack, compress, and elevate. (Fig. 11–5). This will control blood flow and reduce swelling of tissue. Fluoromethane vasocoolant spray is used on the skin for a rapid cooling effect (see Fig. 8–7). It evaporates quickly and acts as an anaesthetic, which is useful for trigger point therapy and for stretching the muscles.

   Caution: Avoid overuse. It may freeze the skin.

For Burns. Cold and ice water bags help to slow the burning and help to heal the injured area. Immerse the burn site in water if the skin is unbroken.

To Reduce Fever. Use tepid or cold water to lower and remove the heat from a body.

Caution. Do not use cryotherapy for extended periods (15 to 20 minutes is suggested). Sports massage therapy suggests 5 minutes on, 5 minutes off. Do not use on persons with depressed sensitivity to temperature (**paresthesia**), coronary artery disease, paralysis, diabetes, certain rheumatoid conditions, debility, and chill. Do not put frozen gel packs directly on the skin.

   As soon as cold or ice application is removed, a more lasting effect on the body takes place:

- Skin returns to warmed and relaxed state.
- Circulation increases.
- Nerve sensitivity increases.
- Adjacent body cells are stimulated; function is improved.
- Feeling of well-being is experienced.

Use of Heat or Warmth

For Toxin Removal. Immersion in a long, hot bath, steam room, or sauna stimulates the excretion of toxins from the body. It induces sweating. (See Box 11–4 for the

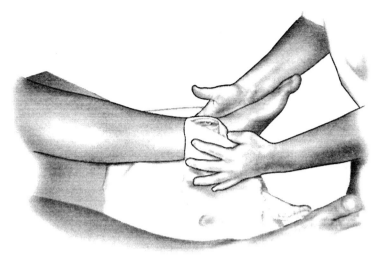

A

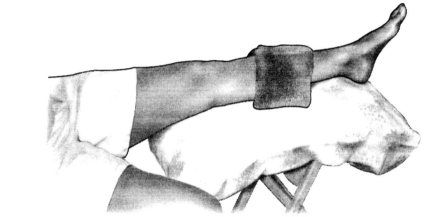

B

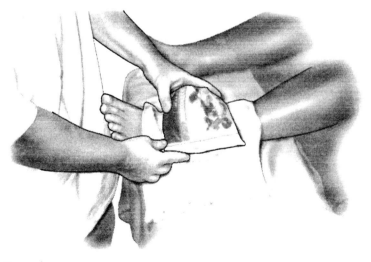

C

FIGURE 11–5. Use of various techniques for cryotherapy. **A.** Iced soda can. **B.** Iced flax seed-filled pillow. **C.** Frozen vegetables from freezer.

BOX 11–4   IMMEDIATE EFFECTS OF USE OF HEAT OR WARMTH

- Warms the skin; relaxes it, causes sweating.
- Increase circulation; blood is brought to the surface of the skin. Tepid saline bath is excellent for this.
- Increases leucocyte migration.
- Increases inflammation through heat and more blood entering the area.
- Increases metabolism; speeds up action of the area.
- Decreases pain; calms and relaxes the area.
- Decreases tissue stiffness and muscle spasms; softens connective tissue. Relaxes muscles and connective tissue.

---

immediate effects of the use of heat and warmth.) Epsom salts and common salt baths aid the removal of toxins and reduce cramps and muscle spasms. Compresses can be used locally as well.

Caution. If a client lives alone or is not in general good health, modify the use of hydrotherapy techniques to those the client may use safely. Check water temperature before getting into the bath. Check wrist pulse before and during the bath. If the client complains of unpleasant reactions, remove him or her from the water and place cold compresses on the forehead and/or the back of the neck. It is important that a client rest following any hydrotherapy session. A massage following the hydrotherapy treatment is an excellent combination for treatment and rest.

Contrast Applications

- Dilates and constricts the local arteries, arterioles, and capillaries alternately.
- Increases circulation and venous flow.
- Moves metabolites and increases tissue feeling.
- Decreases edema.
- Used in subacute conditions for stimulation of total body healing.

Caution. In contrast application, the use of cold is more penetrating than the application of heat, and generally the time is less for the cold application. Examples are hot water, 3 to 5 minutes; cold water, 30 seconds to 2 minutes. Always repeat the alternating of hot and cold water at least three times, finishing with cold water. Do not use for persons with decreased skin sensitivity to temperature (paresthesia). Do not use for acute conditions, for vascular diseases, on persons with hypertension, or on persons with metal implants.

BOX 11-5   RICE

- **R**est is needed for regeneration and healing to occur.
- **I**ce reduces metabolism, therefore lessening secondary injury, keeping the processes of the body from making the injury worse.
- **C**ompression helps control edema by promoting absorption of fluids that pool at the injury site.
- **E**levation reduces blood and fluid flow to the injured area. Less throbbing will also aid reduction of pain.

RICE—First Aid

RICE is an acronym for rest, ice, compression, and elevation (Box 11–5). It is the recipe for acute soft tissue injuries such as sprains and strains. Always refer serious injury to a physician. The treatment reduces damage to the area concerned, decreases pain, and muscle spasm, and therefore reduces total healing time as well as secondary tissue damage caused by the inflammation process (Fig. 11–6).

Sports injuries in particular are treated with RICE. An ice bag is commonly used at athletic events for ice. At home, a plastic bag with ice can be used as well as a bag of frozen green peas or corn. The cold should be applied on the affected part for no longer than 15 to 20 minutes for each application. Five minutes on and five minutes off is another suggested timing for ice.

Do not treat a severe injury without first getting an evaluation by a physician.

After 24 to 48 hours, massage can begin on the area as the client will allow.

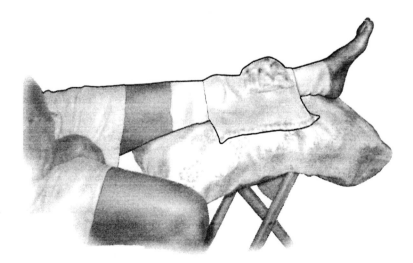

FIGURE 11–6. Use of RICE (Rest, ice, compression, elevation) for first aid.

Thalassotherapy

Thalassotherapy is the use of the sea and sea products, such as seaweed and mud (fango), to add to your use of hydrotheraphy. Many of the major cosmetic companies produce lines of sea products for individual use.

▪ COMPONENTS FOR ADAPTING MASSAGE TO SPECIFIC TREATMENTS

There are various standard components included in every treatment that a therapist performs. The therapist does an assessment and health history on each client, develops the goals and aims for the treatment, gets informed consent from the client, and determines if there are any contraindications. The massage treatment is performed with any hydrotherapy needed. Remedial exercises follow, along with any self-care suggestions for the client. The results of the treatment are recorded in the client's case history file.

However, when dealing with specific ailments, it is important that certain other components be added. The condition must be understood, what causes it, what the outcomes will be, the signs and symptoms, the therapist's aims in the treatment, and the techniques and modalities necessary for treatment and self-care—all are needed. If inflammation is present, modification of treatment may be necessary. Testing must be done and specific techniques introduced specific to the degree of the injury. Therefore, the following section on specific treatments has been included. It is not meant to be an all-inclusive study. Rather, it is an introduction to the therapist of techniques for use in dealing with injuries. Please see Appendix F for a listing of more extensive reference books on assessment and treatment. Selected conditions have been chosen as those most likely to be seen by a massage therapist. They are not in any particular order.

▪ SPECIFIC TREATMENTS

Strains

Partial to total tearing of the muscle due to injury.

Three Classifications

- First degree: up to 20 percent tear
- Second degree: 20 to 75 percent tear
- Third degree: 75 percent to complete tear

Causes. Sudden movement, overuse, violent contraction, repeated minor trauma, unprepared for activity.

Observations. Assess injury site and distal tissue for swelling and color change, check client's face for pain and fear, check gait.

Palpation. Palpate the affected area for tenderness, indentations in the tissue, or contour alteration of tissue. Assess inflammation. Test the joints crossed by the affected muscle.

Short-Term Treatment Goals. Reduce inflammation, increase lymphatic draining, increase circulation. Decrease pain, spasms, and hypertonicity. Maintain ROM without increased injury.

Long-Term Treatment Goals. Restore healthy tissue, restore function, eliminate adhesions, reduce compensations.

Hydrotherapy. RICE in initial stages, ice, contrast baths. If chronic, deep, moist heat, frictioning of scar and ice.

Massage. Treat proximal to site to increase drainage and circulation and reduce hypertonicity. Treat unaffected limb for compensations. In the acute stage, use lymph node pumping, light stroking, and vibration proximally. Rocking and shaking may be used. Golgi tendon organ (GTO) release of affected muscle.

Early Subacute Stages. Use Swedish massage to relax the muscles of the involved area, and proximal drainage, distal lymphatic and circulation work to heal tissue. When scar tissue forms, use frictioning, passive resistive ROM, and stretching.

Chronic. To reduce adhesions, restore full usage, treat compensations, use deep frictioning and contrast-relax stretches.

Client Self-Care. Hydrotherapy, self-massage, remedial exercise.

Length of Treatment

- First degee: 1 week.
- Second degree: 1 to 2 weeks.
- Third degree: 3 or more weeks.

Treat 1 to 2 times a week, 1/2-hour treatments. Decrease frequency as progress occurs.

Sprains

Joint injury and/or bone misalignment that causes ligaments, joint capsules, and tendons to be stretched unduly. They may also be torn.

Three classifications. Same as for strains.

Causes. Sudden, violent twist or torque or bending beyond normal ROM (may be compromised by arthritis, postural misalignments, and loose ligaments).

Observations. Same as for strains.

Palpation. Same as for strains. Test the joints crossed by the affected ligaments.

Short-Term Treatment Goals. RICE treatment in initial stages. Decrease inflammation, decrease edema, increase lymphatic drainage, maintain ROM, reduce formation of scar tissue.

Long-Term Treatment Goals. Restore ROM, avoid compensatory changes.

Hydrotherapy. RICE therapy 24 to 48 hours. If chronic, deep moist heat to soften adhesions and increase circulation. Transverse friction to injured ligaments with ROM will help functional scar tissue form for proper alignment of an injury site.

Massage. If moderate to severe, refer to physician. Treat unaffected limb to reduce compensations. Massage proximal areas; lymphatic drainage; gliding, and kneading to prevent spasms, muscle stripping, and GTO releases.

- Acute stage. Use lymphatic node pumping: light gliding towards the heart. Avoid distal work. Passive, pain-free ROM.
- Subacute stage. As inflammation subsides, begin to prevent adhesions. Gentle cross-fiber friction to ligament, distal vibrations, and gentle muscle squeezing.
- Chronic stage. Treat connective tissue restrictions; proximal lymphatic drainage, reduce scar tissue, do frictioning, and use ice.

Client Self-Care. Hydrotherapy, self-massage, and remedial exercise.

Length of Treatment

- First degree: 4 to 5 days.
- Second degree: 7 to 10 days.
- Third degree: 2 to 3 weeks.

Short, frequent treatments to begin; lengthen treatments as healing progresses.

Bursitis

Inflammation of a bursa, which is a small sac lined with synovial fluid found near joints. Bursitis is often secondary to an injury or a postural deviation. It is a compression injury. Common sites for bursitis are subacromial bursitis in the shoulder (Fig. 11–7) and retrocalcaneal bursitis in the heel.

Causes. Low-grade infection in the joint, dislocation, tendonitis, bacterial infection, gout, or arthritis. Sometimes calcium deposits in joints irritate bursae through overuse and repetitive movements, which are usually occupationally induced.

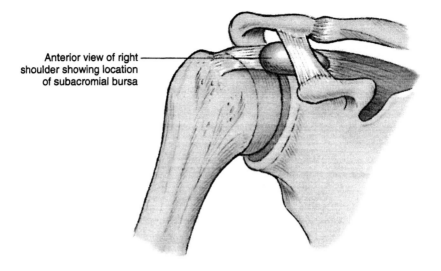

Anterior view of right — shoulder showing location of subacromial bursa

FIGURE 11–7. Location of subacromial bursitis.

Observations. Check for local swelling at bursa site. Watch client's face for pain. Assess posturally once pain is gone.

Palpation. Check for heat and swelling, excessive fluid, and hypertonic muscles as well as pain when compressed. Test the joints and compare bilaterally. Sometimes a "painful arc" of movement will be noted. The pain may start after movement is started. Pain will cease someplace in ROM and finish pain free. Treat the muscles affecting the movement in the "painful area."

Signs and Symptoms. Acute stages last 48 to 72 hours. Intense pain can affect sleep. Inflammation is present. Will last 10 days and then fade away. The chronic stage can last for years. Pain is present. Tissue feels "boggy" and there is swelling.

Short-Term Treatment Goals. Decrease inflammation and pain. Reduce muscle spasms and trigger points (TP). Decrease sympathetic nervous system reaction. Rest is needed and sometimes anti-inflammatory medication helps.

Long-Term Treatment Goals. Prevent recurrence, reduce compensation, find cause, and do postural assessment necessary. If the offending activity is stopped, the bursa will usually return to a normal state.

Hydrotherapy. Acute stage, ice; chronic stage, heat to surrounding area, not on the bursa. Contrast baths.

Massage. The benefits of massage are indirect here. Massage opposite limb to reduce hypertonicity. Relaxing massage to decrease sympathetic nervous system control. Massage the entire area to help normalize all muscles in the area.

- Acute stage. Rest and elevate. No massage on site.
- Subacute stage. Lymphatic drainage, proximal work. Do not compress bursae. Lift tissue.
- Chronic stage. When inflammation reduces, glide and scoop around bursae, ROM, friction adhesions, and ice.

Client Self-Care. Rest from cause, relaxation techniques. Free-swimming limb exercises. If chronic, warm site and hydrotherapy. For flare-ups, use contrast baths. Ice and rest.

Length of Treatment. Twice times a week, 1/2-hour each time. Decrease to once a week as healing progresses.

Fibromyalgia or Fibrositis Syndrome

Diffuse musculoskeletal pain and tenderness in specific points. Sleep may be affected, morning stiffness, tingling, numbness, anxiety, and depression. Functional gastrointestinal and urinary tract irritation. Aggravated by stress, cold, overexertion. Women are more affected than men. Lack of sleep, postural misalignments, and hyperlordosis may be causes. Related conditions are migraines, irritable bowel or bladder syndrome, and chronic fatigue syndrome.

Treatment Goals. Relaxation and stress reduction. Gentle Swedish massage; day-to-day fluctuations occur, so adjust the treatment to the client's condition at each session. Avoid lengthy treatments.

Hydrotherapy. Warm baths.

Self-Care. Mild exercise. May be painful for 6 to 8 weeks.

Bell's Palsy

Facial paralysis that affects cranial nerve VII; usually unilateral. Thought to be caused by a cycle of edema and compressive ischemia of nerve in the narrow facial canal of the temporal bone. Colds and chills can trigger it, as can stress factors. Sometimes dental surgery, inner ear infections, or direct trauma are related to the condition. There are also correlations to pregnancy, diabetes, and hypertension.

Signs and Symptoms. Inability to raise the corner of the mouth; loss of blinking reflex in the eye; unable to wrinkle forehead, eye cannot close, eye weeps; unable to dilate nostril, unable to move food from affected side of mouth; dropping of cheek on affected side of face.

Massage. Gentle, light Swedish strokes applied to the face; trigger point (TP) therapy from chin to ear and across forehead. Massage should be done daily, and then more infrequently as nerve strength returns.

Client Self-Care. Daily exercises of all normal activities. Example include smiling, whistling, and puckering lips.

Outcome. If treatment begins immediately and is maintained, it is likely that the client will have near 100 percent recovery over time. Exercises are extremely important to return functions. Vitamin B_{12} injections and corticosteroid drug therapy are effective and can shorten recovery time.

Sciatic Nerve Lesion and Piriform Syndrome

Loss of enervation of the muscles that dorsiflex the ankle and evert the foot. (L4 to S3 areas may be affected.) "Drop foot" may result. Can be caused by trauma, accidents, fractures, hip replacement surgery, dislocation of the hip, gunshot wounds, previous injections to gluteals, and compression to nerve roots due to degenerative disc disease. These injuries often mimic symptoms of a lumbar disc protrusion on a spinal nerve. The sciatic nerve runs on top of five deep hip rotators and under the piriform muscle as it leaves the sacral plexus. It travels down the limb. In a small number of cases (15 percent), the sciatic nerve becomes compressed. See Figure 11–8 for site of sciatic nerve and palpation site.

Signs and Symptoms. Look for enervation loss below the knee, all of the foot except instep skin, and medial malleolus. All joints of foot and leg may be affected. Pain may be felt in the gluteal area, down the posterior thigh, and all the way down the leg into the foot. Prolonged sitting aggravates the condition, as does activity that uses the hip extensively.

Assessment. Use the piriform test to see if that muscle and sciatic nerve are involved. The piriform test is performed as follows. Position the client at the edge of a table, in a side-lying position, with the affected hip presented. Bring the femoral head into medial rotation, stabilize the pelvis, and apply gentle pressure downward on the knee to stretch the piriform muscle. Keep the pelvis vertical and do not allow the client to twist the torso. If additional pain is felt, it is likely caused by the piriform muscle and a compressed sciatic nerve (Fig. 11–9).

Further testing might include muscle testing of the surrounding area to identify strains or spasms. Rest, anti-inflammatory medication, stretching, and strengthening once the pain is reduced are indicated.

Massage. Perform massage, side-lying the client to avoid compression and traction on the nerve. Pillows may be used to prop the client for comfort. Treat the leg with noncompression strokes. Spread tissue; do not compress. Treat pelvis, back, and neck for any compensation. If edema is present, use lymphatic drainage techniques. As tissue regenerates, more vigorous treatments may be given.

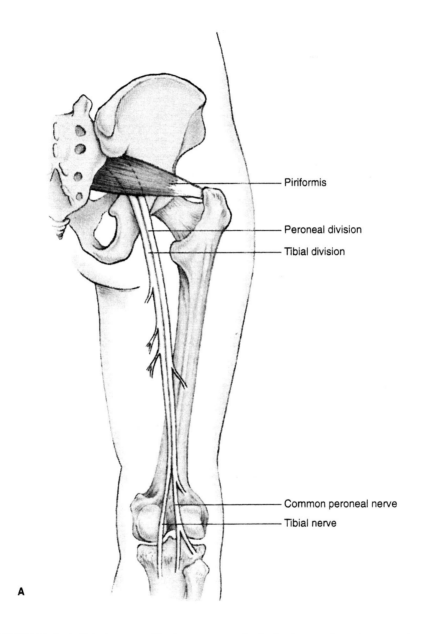

A

FIGURE 11–8. A. Sciatic nerve. The longest nerve in the body sometimes becomes impinged by the piriform muscle and can cause pain down the entire leg. *(Continued)*

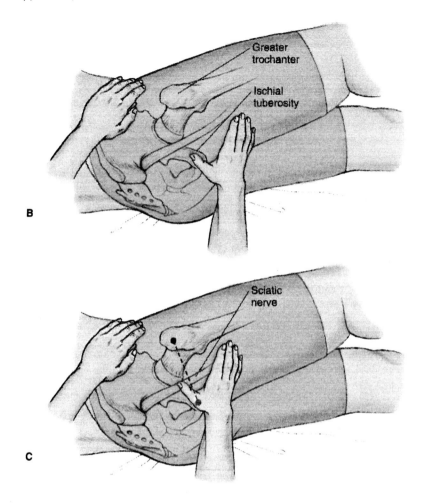

FIGURE 11–8 (cont.). B. Greater trochanter and ischial tuberosity. **C.** Palpation of sciatic nerve. In a side-lying position, the sciatic nerve can be located halfway between the ischial tuberosity and the greater trochanter.

After pain is gone, client can begin to pick up small articles with the toes. Recovery time on peripheral nerves is slow—a rate of 1 to 3 mm daily. Watch for antagonist muscle contracture and treat as well. Massage can also help prevent spasming.

Do not use hydrotherapy in this case, because the client may not be able to sense temperatures correctly and nerve tissue is very fragile. Deep transverse friction will help create functional scarring. In paralysis, work joints and keep them in good health. Proprioceptive neuromuscular facilitation (PNF) treatment is also good. Keeping the client's morale high is most important.

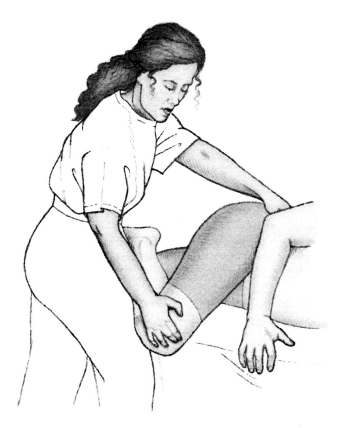

FIGURE 11–9. Piriform test technique to examine for impingement of the sciatic nerve by the piriform muscle.

Whiplash

Rapid movement of the head, especially in flexion and extension (usually sustained in car accidents), results in a combination of injuries affecting the muscles, ligaments, vertebrae, nerves, fasciae, and blood vessels of the cervical region of the spine. Pain and muscle spasm may not occur for several days after the accident.

Often, a physician will prescribe massage for such an injury. Keep excellent records for this client, as lawsuits are often involved. Sometimes the massage therapist is one of a team of healthcare professionals treating this client. You may need to confer with the others as the case progresses. The therapists needs to have an excellent understanding of the anatomy of this area as well as the specific muscles involved for ROM.

Health History. Get an assessment by a physician. Question the client as to complete details on accidents and health prior to this accident.

Observations. Notice any compensations. Do postural analysis, especially of the head, neck, and trunk.

Palpation. Look for tenderness, edema, inflammation, spasming, trigger points. Sometimes, all of the neck muscles may be involved in some way.

Testing. May be painful. If x-rays or a radiology report are available, ask to see them. Your referring physician can clarify what you are seeing on x-rays. If possible, do passive ROM tests and manual resistive tests as well.

Signs and Symptoms. Usually present themselves sometime after the accident occurs. Signs and symptoms include pain, inflammation, difficulty swallowing, muscle spasms, hypertonicity, numbness or tingling, headaches, temporomandibular joint dysfunction, chest pains, back pain, nausea, shortness of breath, earache, pain while chewing, and reduced ROM of the cervical spine.

Short-Term Treatment Goals. Reduce pain, edema, spasming, inflammation, and trigger point. Maintain ROM, prevent adhesions. Refer the client to a physician if he or she has not been evaluated. Whiplash may involve spinal nerve injury or spinal cord injury as well. Applications of cold and rest will aid pain and spasming.

Long-Term Treatment Goals. Strengthen weak muscles, increase ROM, reduce compensatory changes. Treat accompanying dysfunctions such as temporomandibular joint dysfunction. Trigger point. After the acute phase, heat may give pain relief and aid relaxation.

Hydrotherapy

- Acute. Cold or ice.
- Subacute. Contrast applications, whirlpool or showers.
- Chronic. Hydrocollator or hot moist heat. If in pain, do not use weight on neck. Use hot bath instead.

Massage. Securely pillow the neck or do seated massage. Gentle techniques, careful ROM or none, depending on client's anxiety level. Treat whole body (seatbelt injury, for example); relaxation techniques, lots of rest, and breathing exercises may be suggested. Use broad, long strokes of Swedish massage but no percussion to increase circulation. Focus on relaxing the client. Use lymphatic drainage techniques and cranial–sacral techniques. As health returns to area, deeper massage may be done and deep muscle stripping and TP work is indicated. Fascial techniques on the whole neck are also indicated, along with passive ROM, contraction–relaxation, and stretching.

Client Self-Care. Remedial exercises; passive stretching and head to chin tucks. Hydrotherapy as needed. Avoid long, continuous wearing of support collars if the physician agrees.

Length of Treatment. Varies from a few weeks to months. Three times a week to start, 1/2-hour treatments; then 1 to 2 times a week. Reassess periodically.

Carpal Tunnel Syndrome

Medial nerve compression syndrome located on the anterior region of the wrist. A tunnel is formed by the soft tissue retinaculum on the anterior and the carpal bones on the posterior. The tendons of the hand, the flexor muscles, and the nerves of the hand run through the tunnel.

Causes. Overuse and repetitive motion are often the causes of muscle swelling and compression on the medial nerve, causing pain and numbness and loss of ROM. The lateral 3½ digits may be involved. See Figure 11–10 for site of carpal tunnels.

Observations. A good health history is essential and will usually show overuse and repetitive motion of the finger and hand flexor muscles. Pain will often be localized in the anterior wrist and the palmar surface of the hand. The second, third, and

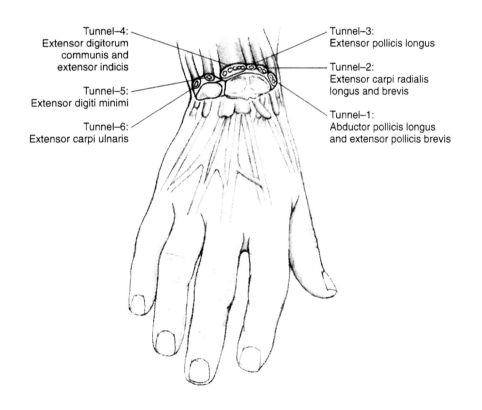

FIGURE 11–10. Carpal tunnels along the dorsum of the wrist transport extensor tendons to the hand.

fourth fingers may also be affected. Lack of grip strength, motor weakness, numbness, parasthesia, and edema may be present.

Testing. Perform Phalen's test and look for Tinel's sign. *Phalen's test* is as follows. Client places both wrists together flexed to the maximum degree, with the dorsal surfaces of the hands touching, for 1 minute. If this produces pain or tingling, carpal tunnel syndrome may be present (Fig. 11–11A).

For *Tinel's sign*, supinate the client's hand and arm and lightly tap on the anterior surface of the wrist. If this produces pain that follows the median nerve distribution, it is likely to indicate carpal tunnel syndrome (Fig. 11–11B). Check also for

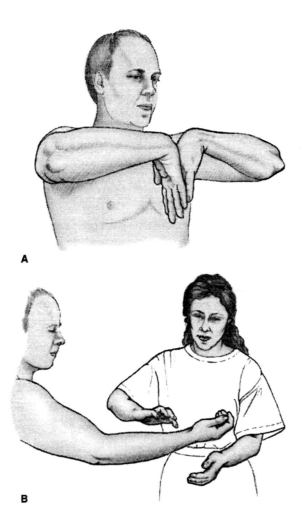

A

B

FIGURE 11–11. A. Phalen's test, used to examine for carpal tunnel syndrome. **B.** Tinel's sign. *(Continued)*

loss of strength and weakness in the thenar. Also, check sleeping patterns, if appropriate to the client.

In the *Finkelstein test*, the client makes a fist, tucking the thumb inside the other fingers, stabilizing the forearm with one hand and deviates the wrist to the ulnar side. If the client feels a sharp pain in the area of the tunnel, there is a strong evidence of stenosing tenosynovitis (Fig. 11–11C).

Short-Term Treatment. Rest from activity and decrease inflammation by the use of ice and/or anti-inflammatory medication. Massage is useful in decreasing tension in the flexor muscles of the wrist and in softening fascia to reduce pain.

Long-Term Treatment. When pain allows, deep stripping of the muscles is effective in removing accumulated toxins and unsticking fascia. Arms, shoulders, and neck

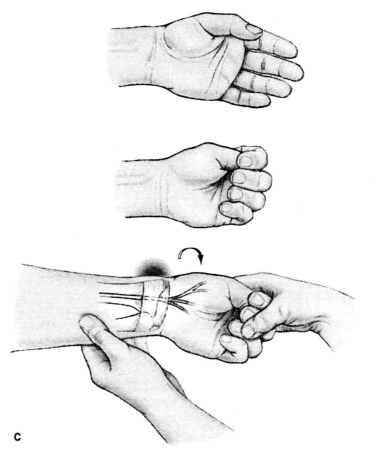

c

FIGURE 11–11 (cont.). C. Finkelstein test.

should also be massaged, as referred pain travels up the arm to the neck and shoulders. Help the client in terms of self-massage and alleviating repetitive motions as prevention methods.

Massage. Swedish massage, myofascial release, and neuromuscular techniques can all be used as pain allows. If the therapist is not successful in reducing pain and inflammation, refer the client to a physician. Sometimes, surgery is needed. If overuse is not reduced, the condition may return again, even after surgery.

Often, the medical community will suggest injections of corticosteroid to reduce inflammation, and medications and surgery to relieve the pressure on the nerve for those unresponsive clients.

Plantar Fascitis

The longitudinal arch area of the foot becomes irritated and an inflammation of the plantar fascia results. Once the plantar fascia is shortened, it becomes stressed and stuck. Pain and intense itching is often felt at the calcaneous attachment of the fascia. If severe, this condition often involves ossification and bone spurs at the attachment. Improper biomechanics of legs and feet may be involved.

Signs and Symptoms. Pain along the bottom of the foot, especially when active. Intense itching and a pulling sensation along the length of the plantar fascia from the metatarsal heads at the distal plantar fascia attachment sites to the anterior calcaneous attachment. Tenderness, redness, and pain, or swelling, may be felt along the entire arch area. Check the gastrocnemius muscle for tightness. Prolonged standing and walking may also be the cause.

Treatment Goals. Rest, limited activity, stretching of the Achilles tendon and flexor muscles of the foot. Reduce pain and inflammation. Cryotherapy and/or contrast hydrotherapy treatments. Elimination of adhesions, restoration of full muscle length, and proper biomechanics to prevent recurrence.

Massage. Myofascial spreading techniques, reflexology, and Swedish massage to the bottom of the foot may unstick and spread fascia and soften tissue as well as relax it. Deep longitudinal stripping will also elongate the fibers. Stretching the gastrocnemius and plantar fascia is best done by the client as self-care. Rest and hydrotherapy may also be done by the client at home.

Tendonitis

Because tendons do not stretch readily, inflammation of a tendon often occurs when it is subjected to a force beyond its capabilities. This can occur when a sudden force exerts pressure or when chronic stress is repeated over and over again. Microtearing often results as well as tendon ruptures. Scarring within the tendon may result and pain occurs.

Cause. Microtearing of individual fibers in the tendon due to repeated stress. Sometimes a small piece of bone may tear away as the tendon ruptures (avulsion fracture). Surgical repair may be needed for tendon repairs, depending on their severity. Examples of this injury include Achilles tendonitis, elbow tendonitis (tennis elbow), golfers' elbow, and bicipital tendonitis. Limited blood supply in tendons may prolong the healing process.

Testing and Palpation. Assess for tenderness, trigger points, and pain in the involved muscles and joints, and isolate the affected areas. Note muscle weakness. Do all testing and palpation bilaterally to note any differences.

For the *tennis elbow test,* client is sitting or standing. Support the lateral elbow region with one hand with the thumb over the tendons of the wrist extensor muscles. Hold the wrist in 45-degree extension. Still holding the wrist, try to bring the wrist into flexion. While doing so, press on the extensor tendons of the wrist with the thumb. If pain is caused, it is likely that some epicondylitis is present.

For the *golfer's elbow test,* client is sitting or standing. One hand is on the medial elbow region with thumb over flexor tendons of the wrist. The other hand is over the client's palm (palm in 20 to 30 degrees of hyperextension). While holding in this position, the therapist tries to extend the wrist further while pressing on the flexor tendons just distal to the medial epicondyle of the humerus. If pain occurs, medial epicondylitis is likely.

In the *bicipital tendinitis test,* or Speed's test, the client is standing with shoulder flexed to 90 degrees, elbow extended, palm supine. While client holds this position, the therapist pushes the distal portion of the lower arm downward. Anterior shoulder pain indicates likely bicipital tendon involvement (Fig. 11–12).

Short-Term Treatment Goals. Determine ROM limitations and possible repetitive motions causing the injury. Reduce pain and inflammation. Rest is needed, but not immobilization. This will lead to adhesions. Hydrotherapy (cold) and anti-inflammatory medication may be used.

Long-Term Treatment Goals. Stretching of the involved tendon to develop functional scar tissue, several times a day. Reduction in tension of area's muscles to reduce referred pain. Increase ROM and prevention of recurrence. Self-care exercises, hydrotherapy, and massage as the site of injury allows.

Massage. Gentle Swedish massage and myofascial release will reduce tension and soften tissue in the area, as soon as pain allows. Deep transverse friction on tendons will break up fibrous adhesions and help to align tissue. Cold applications of hydrotherapy will reduce pain before and after massage. Stripping of muscles will help restore balance in the muscles of the area and help decrease the mechanical loading on the tendon that causes the microtearing.

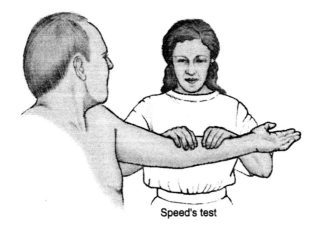

Speed's test

FIGURE 11–12. Speed's test, which examines for bicipital tendonitis. Pain is often felt at the tendon of the head of the biceps brachia.

▪ SPECIAL POPULATIONS

Specialization in massage has occurred just as it has in medicine in general. As the field expands and more modalities are created, it is impossible to be efficient in everything. One way to decide on a specialization is to identify a population in society with which you would like to work. To this aim, this section of this chapter is devoted to special populations in our society today.

Pregnancy and Infant Massage

Pregnancy and infant massage has grown out of the intertwined needs of both the mother and the infant child. During pregnancy, the mother has physiological, psychological, emotional, and spiritual needs in connection with the growing child within her. She feels a need to make a connection with her child. Although abdominal massage is not recommended in the first trimester (1 to 3 months), a general Swedish massage is indicated to reduce or remove stress and tension brought on by this new commitment in her life. After the first 3 months, abdominal massage can be added to the routine so as to encourage the bonding and union between the mother and her unborn child. The emotional health and stability of both will be enhanced. As the child grows in the womb, the mother may experience low back pain as well as general stress and tension. Massage as you would normally—with the adaptations that will now be described.

Positioning. Position the client where she is comfortable. In the first few months, the prone position and the supine position may be used with extra support under the back and bended knees. Do not use these positions in the second half of pregnancy. Use the side-lying position, propping pillows where needed for support and comfort. The body support system may also be used.

Contraindications to massage during pregnancy include high blood pressure and excess edema. Refer to a physician as special conditions such as pre-eclampsia and toxemia can sometimes be present. Avoid varicose veins. Go around them, using light pressure in the massage.

If the massage therapist has been trained in pregnancy and infant massage (see Appendix F for additional material), he or she may accompany the soon-to-be mother to the hospital or birthing center and massage her between contractions. (Be sure to have the doctor's or the midwife's permission.)

After the birth, both mother and child will benefit from massage (Fig. 11–13). Often, the massage therapist will teach the new mother to massage her own infant, thus aiding the bonding between the two as well as greatly aiding the infant's development.

Athletes

Sports massage therapy is a blend of Russian techniques modified by Western Swedish techniques. The Russians perfected sports massage about 15 years ago, says Dr. Michael Yessi, editor of *Soviet Sports Review Journal*. Every Russian team now has a sports massage therapist assigned to it and the therapist travels with the team to every competition.

Soon the Europeans and the Americans both were interested in sports massage. Even the New York Giants sent Johnny Parker, one of their coaches, to Russia to investigate. They won the Super Bowl the year they started to use the techniques.

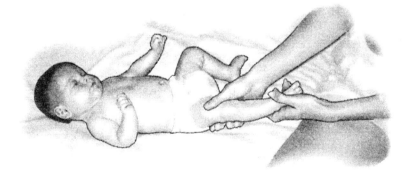

FIGURE 11–13. Infant massage has been proven to be most beneficial for the infant in the areas of metabolism, growth and development, and bonding.

Now many teams have massage therapists who travel with their team. The American Massage Therapy Association has certified sports massage therapists, many of whom will be working at each Olympics to be held in the future. In 1984, massage was made available to all competing athletes.

Sports massage is divided into three phases: pre-event, before an athlete's competition or before a workout; postevent, after a competition or workout; and rehabilitation, after an injury.

Pre-event massage is aimed at getting the athlete in top form for the next event. It helps prevent injury and it warms the tissue before the event to help maximize performance. There are three basic strokes:

1. Kneading and compression, used pre- or postevent on muscle bellies.
2. Direct pressure, applied with thumb, finger, or elbow to trigger points on tight and tender areas.
3. Light tapotement, to stimulate the muscle.

Sometimes a fourth move, shaking and jostling, is used to release tension.

Postevent massage is used to relax the tired muscle, reduce any spasms or tight spots, and assess any damage. Components of postevent massage are (1) lifting and broadening, (2) compression, and (3) stretching.

Rehabilitation or restorative massage is used during training and between competitions to restore an injured athlete to good physical condition so that he or she may again compete. It helps restore mobility and flexibility to injured tissue, reduces recovery time, and may extend the athlete's career. The components of rehabilitation are assessment, short- and long-term treatment goals, hydrotheraphy, massage, and exercise.

Elderly and Chronically Ill

The elderly can greatly benefit from massage, but certain precautions and adjustments should be made to general massage practices. Bones are more brittle, not as flexible, and apt to break. Joints are worn down from use and some form of arthritis is likely. Muscles are less toned and have decreased, having been replaced by connective tissue and fat. The trunk tends to collapse during aging, and circulation to the extremities may have lessened. Many elderly are on medications.

Also, many elderly are alone, their spouses gone and their families busy. Everyone needs touching and caring, but the elderly more so. Also, finances are usually tight. Many massage therapists adjust their fees and increase their time spent at a treatment, as many elderly want and need to talk.

The elderly in rest homes and nursing homes need massage too, but because of low finances and being tucked away, they often receive minimum touching, few visitors, and no massage. If you are affiliated with a school, why not volunteer your time to give a massage to such a cause. Many schools have outreach projects in which students are accompanied by an instructor and given time for their massage even if it ends up being just holding hands with an elderly person and listening to old stories (Fig. 11–14).

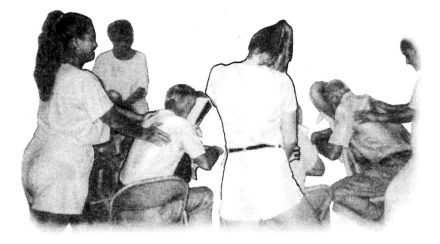

FIGURE 11–14. Massage in a nursing home.

General Instructions. Proceed cautiously. Get a good health history if possible. Get lots of feedback from the client and focus your intention so that you are giving 100 percent of yourself in a loving, caring way.

Persons who have a debilitating disease such as Parkinson's disease, lupus, rheumatoid arthritis, multiple sclerosis, AIDS, or chronic fatigue syndrome may show very slow signs of recovery or, in fact, their condition may be deteriorating.

Massage can help in the short term but not in the long term. Life with a chronic disease is no fun for anyone concerned. It is frustrating and hard to deal with whether you are the patient or the caregiver. Even if a return to health is indicated, it takes a long time and a great deal of commitment by everyone concerned. Massage can help the patient to reduce the stress connected with the disease. It can provide a time "away" from the disease. It can help the person relax. It can also empower him or her to take control of the disease, not let it take control of them.

Massage and hydrotherapy, if indicated, should be designed for the client visit by visit, as the disease may fluctuate day by day. Clients who are chronically ill are usually under a physician's care and taking medications. Check with the physician before starting any massage program. Ask about the effects of the disease and the medications and how massage may affect the client. Learn all you can about the disease so that you may help the client as much as you can.

If the client is interested, alternative approaches may also be used, including relaxation techniques, spiritual healing, affirmation and visualization, and behavior modification, among others. Certainly, discovering all there is to know about a disease is the first step. Then, discovery of the writings of people like Dr. Bernie Siegel, Dr. DeePak Chopra, and others can encourage the client to take inner control and to make the quality of life the best it can be for him or her.

Terminally Ill

Often, in the final years of life, the body has reached a point at which it cannot recover to a healthy state. At this point the client would be under a physician's care. The diagnosis might be cancer, AIDS, complications of a disease such as diabetes, or an assortment of ailments determined to be very slow to improve or terminal. Keeping the patient comfortable in day-to-day living is the aim.

Attitudes about dying differ and the worries associated with death are many. The person feels pain—real or that of separation from loved ones, the loneliness associated with it, and/or any suffering that might accompany it. Some, however, welcome death as a relief and freedom from the cares of this world.

Massage therapists who wish to work with the terminally ill need to make contact with a hospice group and explore the possibilities of massage for the patients in their care. They often have a good volunteer program and offer training for those volunteers.

Massage can still offer much caring, loving, and concern to the terminally ill patient and to those who care for him or her. This is a teamwork situation, as the massage therapist will be one of many caring for the patient. The massage itself would be aimed at relaxation and providing care and concern. It is a different experience for the therapist, who must see the patient decline, die, and then mourn and grieve afterwards. If massage is undertaken, the client in this situation should maintain as much control as possible over the massage.

Disabled, Addiction, and Trauma Victims

If the disabled person has no condition that might be considered a contraindication to massage, massage may be given, with techniques adapted to the individual.

If the client is bedridden, the therapist needs to think of ways to alter body mechanics to protect his or her back. Kneeling or sitting may be considered. Other considerations about treatment time, pressure, and areas of the body to avoid may be needed.

Using massage as part of an addiction program for rehabilitation is a powerful detoxifying tool for healing. However, treatment should be given in the rehabilitation facility as part of an overall program and under the supervision of the medical staff. Response to massage can be unpredictable in these cases and should not be attempted outside these parameters.

Trauma victims, too, may benefit from massage, as it helps to clear the tissues of toxins and memories associated with the trauma. Again, individual needs of the trauma victim will dictate massage treatments as well as possible need of auxillary services such as a psychotherapist, medical specialist, or community support groups.

▪ CASE STUDIES

1. Some years ago my daughter, age 28, called from Toronto in the middle of a cold, bitter winter. She had been working very hard as a waitress and had, the day before, gotten chilled coming home from work. She was sobbing. She

had woken up that morning with one side of her face "droopy." She had gone to the emergency room in a nearby hospital. They examined her, gave her condition the name Bell's palsy, and told her to buy a vibrator and use it on her face. She was bewildered and scared. We arranged an emergency air flight and she arrived the next day. Indeed, her face was "droopy." From the eye corners, cheek, and corner of the mouth, one side of the face was dropped. She had little control of anything on that side of her face. We started several times a day massaging the whole face. We did not use hydrotherapy methods, as it has not been found that they do any good. She received several vitamin B_{12} shots as well. After a few days of looking into a mirror every few minutes, she started doing exercises every time she picked up a mirror, trying to make the muscles work. Slowly, the face regained its tone. The last evidence was a slight downward turn of one side of the mouth every time she smiled. This has reduced to being almost invisible as years have passed.

- What are the other possible causes of the signs and symptoms described?
- Devise a massage treatment plan including the massage routine and client self-care exercises.

2. Diane was a 57-year-old, athletic-type cancer patient receiving postsurgery care and being massaged at an osteopath's office. She had recently had a mastectomy and could not lift her affected arm nor pick anything up. The arm was very edemic and about twice the size of the other arm. She had been told the risk of the cancer metastasizing and understood it, but felt she could not live with her arm, underarm, and shoulder the way it was. She wanted to be active again. The doctor prescribed massage for the whole trunk and neck three times a week to start, to be re-evaluated in 4 weeks. Diane had not looked at her scarring and was afraid to do so. She was just finished with her radiation and worked around her schedule of no massage 3 days before and 3 days after the radiation. The scarring under her arm was like someone had cut a pie into several wedges. Everything was a jumble and not much was in its right place, with muscle and lymph nodes gone. The scarring over the breast area was better, but beginning to contract and get hard. Massage began immediately, although progress was slow, due to tenderness and Diane's need to talk and cry. After 4 weeks, Diane could raise the arm to shoulder level and pick up an empty coffee cup. The smell of burnt flesh during each treatment was lessening. The emphasis for a treatment was to reduce stress, reduce pain, reduce edema, and decrease the effects of the scarring. Several weeks into the treatment, Diane brought a small pink razor in and asked me to shave under her arm. She watched the procedure, holding a hand mirror. She progressed steadily and in several months was released from the doctor's care with about 95 percent use of the arm. Five years later Diane died. Her cancer had consumed her. I went to her funeral and cried.

- Discuss a treatment plan that includes the scarring, reduced ROM for the arm, and edema, and that addresses the psychological effects and stress factors to the client as well as the exercises for strength and ROM improvement.

- Suggest components for her recovery in addition to those mentioned.

3. Rhonda, 40, worked in an office, and whenever the stress factor got too much for her, she would come for massage on her low back, hip rotators, and glutes. The tissue on her buttocks was described by her as a "hard, coiled snake." The only thing that worked to "uncoil" it was heavy palmar friction. The therapist would rub hard, Rhonda would cry out in pain, the therapist would leave it, massage elsewhere on her body, and come back again to rub hard. The snake uncoiled slowly.

   Hydrotherapy and ultrasound were also helpful. The doctor prescribed painkillers, which did little. Treatments were 30 to 60 minutes, several times a week; and as the condition subsided, once a week. The office bought her a new chair and a stool for her legs. Now the condition occurs only when she is under a lot of stress.

   - Devise a treatment plan for her visits, including hydrotherapy and ultrasound.
   - Devise a client self-care plan to reduce stress in her life.

4. David, in his mid-40s, is a professional cricketer on an international team. He runs 20 to 30 yards at top speed and fast bowls the ball to the batter. When he throws the ball, his entire body stretches right out. As he was playing one day, he heard a pop behind his knee and he had to be helped off the field. When he came to the therapist 48 hours later, the posterior upper thigh was black and blue where the hamstring muscle had torn and the blood vessels had burst. At first, he received light massage only and ultrasound. After one week, massage began in earnest behind his knee. Every other day he received contrast hydrotherapy and the client massaged the back of the leg himself every day. He still plays cricket, is a radio sportscaster, and swims in the sea every day to keep fit.

   - Devise a treatment plan for this client.
   - Determine how long treatments should be and the length of time for recovery.

5. Elizabeth, in her mid-40s, was diagnosed with multiple sclerosis 10 years ago. She sometimes had back spasms so bad that she could not move. The therapist would see her at her home. The spasms often included her entire back from the top of her shoulders to her hip bones. Lubricant was heat-producing analgesic cream. She was massaged for a while and then would sweat profusely and panic. Deep breathing was a help, but the therapist would have to stop massaging and talk to her about her "fears." The massage often took longer than 1 hour and often would conclude with a cup of tea, the client and therapist resting until spasms would stop. This client is

under a doctor's care, takes medication, looks after her diet, and is still very active. She still has back spasms but only very occasionally.

- Devise a long-term treatment plan for this client.
- How many treatments would be needed?
- Describe any client self-care you think would be helpful.

6. The students of a massage school are going to a local nursing home that takes the chronically ill as well as elderly people not able to look after themselves any longer. Some of the class will do wheelchair patients in the great room while others will fan out into the rooms doing people on their beds.

- Devise a massage for a wheelchair patient (30 minutes long).
- Devise a massage for a chronically ill person who cannot get out of bed.

7. An athlete comes to you with inflammation at the elbow. You suspect, from palpation, that there is a slight tear in the extensor carpi radialis brevis or longus. It hurts on the outside of the elbow and pain sometimes goes down to the forearm. This is a common injury to racketball players, but others who lift heavy objects, wait tables, and scrub floors also get it. The pain grows steadily worse with time as a minute, V-shaped scar forms over the tear and begins to hurt. Often, everyday activity reinjures it, and uneven healing because of the V-shape makes the scarring worsen. Healing time is generally 6 months to 1 year.

- Plan a treatment to include deep massage to the forearm and deep friction to break up the scar tissue. It can be painful.
- Suggest exercises that may help strengthen and stretch the arm. Suggest ice after exercising.
- You may suggest that the client see a physician and receive an injection of corticosteroid in the precise area of injury.

REVIEW QUESTIONS

1. Identify and discuss the general indicators of inflammation and pain and the role they play in certain pathologies.
2. Describe the three stages of inflammation.
3. Describe the pain–spasm–pain cycle.
4. Discuss how massage would be modified and used in the three stages of inflammation.
5. Discuss the three types of pain: acute, chronic, and intractable.
6. Discuss the types of hydrotherapy and what they might be used for: compresses, sprays, baths, steam, body wraps.

7. What are the short- and long-term effects of heat and cold on the body?
8. Describe the use of RICE.
9. What would the short-term treatment goals be for strain?
10. What would the long-term treatment goals be for sprains?
11. What might causes bursitis?
12. Discuss a general treatment plan for Bell's palsy.
13. Discuss the length of time for recovery from a sciatic nerve lesion.
14. Discuss the treatment areas needing massage in a whiplash case.
15. Discuss the adaptations to be made by the therapist in massaging an infant.
16. Name the three basic strokes in sports massage, and discuss when they are used.
17. Describe how massage can be helpful for the chronically ill.
18. Choose one of the case studies at the end of this chapter, and answer the questions at the end of that case study.
19. Define the vocabulary terms at the beginning of this chapter.

CASE STUDIES

How to Use the Case Studies

The case studies presented here are meant to be open-ended. All are real cases; some are composites of several cases. All names have been changed. No treatment is planned, nor is the therapist–client interaction planned. The studies can be used in role-playing or as a starter in class for discussion. Treatment plans can be outlined and, in fact, the actual massage could be given and evaluated. Information not provided can be added by the student, thus making each case different.

- Choose a case and explain how you would work with the client. What additional material do you need? Develop a treatment plan that addresses the client concerns. Perform the massage on a fellow student and ask for an evaluation.
- Choose a case study and decide on a modality other than Swedish massage. How would you approach the client with the idea of a new modality? Plan a treatment, perform it, and get an evaluation.
- Choose a case study and add details so that it becomes a difficult case. How would you approach the client? What modality would you choose and why? Plan your treatment, perform it, and ask for evaluation.

1. Lucille, 65, has a rare blood disease. She has been coming for treatments weekly for 10 years. As long as she has her massage regularly, the disease is kept under control. She is under a physician's care and was referred by her physician to begin the treatments.

2. Joan, 16, was an abused child and was referred for massage as part of her therapy at that time. She comes for therapy now whenever her mother thinks the situation warrants it. Joan does not object.

3. Carol, 38, is an office worker doing computer work. She has low back pain and neck pain often. She has two teenage children and runs a busy household as well. She comes weekly to a student clinic for massage.

4. Mark, 48, is a hairdresser and a massage therapist. He works most days and evenings and, on the weekend, is a runner. He often participates in statewide marathons. His shoulders and arms need attention, but he is physically fit.

5. Diane, 17, is a high school student, very petite and active in school sports. She plays volleyball and participates in cheerleading. Her shoulders and low back often ache and her posture is not good. Her shoulders slouch and are rounded, giving her an "old woman" look.

6. Keith, in his 40s, is a fork-lift operator. He is a big man with massive chest and shoulders but a small waist. He likes to be around people but does not come in for massage unless he is hurting.

7. Theresa, 33, is a new mother. She did not get massage when she was pregnant but did receive a massage as part of the package of services at her birthing center. Now she wants her baby to receive massage and she wants to learn to give the massage herself.

8. Robert, in his mid-30s, does not want to take his clothes off for a massage. He has heard of reflexology and is willing to try it. He has an old ankle injury that sometimes gives him trouble.

9. Jean, 60-ish, has been receiving neuromuscular and Swedish massage for years. She has an old hip and disc injury that flares up from time to time. She had a series of structural alignment treatments a few years ago. She feels something needs to release the hip and is willing to try something new.

10. Your friend speaks to you about his dog, a German shepherd named Joey, who is showing signs of hip dysplegia. Can you do anything for the dog?

11. Serena, 50, strained her back while pulling out a bed to remake it. She is doubled over and you cannot go to her right away. What is she to do? You go to her home later in the day. After several visits, she hurts her back again, this time from pushing a large garden pot with her foot. Her leg is in spasm as well as her back.

12. Randy, 15, is brought to you by his mother. He has scoliosis, as she does. Her back is hurting; his is not. He really doesn't want to be treated, yet his mother wants him to avoid her plight.

13. Angela, age 7, is a small child who has been diagnosed as having cerebral palsy. She cannot walk, but crawls and can sit up without help. Her parents want to see what massage can do for her. She is uncooperative sometimes and does not participate willingly when you massage her. Her parents do not push her. You feel she could be more independent.

14. Rita is a 28-year-old woman with pain in her upper thoracic region and neck. Her hips are uneven; the right hip is high and rotated anteriorly. The glutes are tight. Neck work brings on emotional release. Design a massage treatment using structural alignment and energy work as well.

CODE OF ETHICS

Code of Ethics of the National Certification Board
for Therapeutic Massage and Bodywork

*The Code of Ethics of the National Certification Board for Therapeutic Massage and Bodywork (NCBTMB) specifies professional standards that allow for the proper discharge of the massage therapist and/or bodyworker's responsibilities to those served, that protects the integrity of the profession and safeguards the interest of individual clients.

*Those practitioners Nationally Certified in Therapeutic Massage and Bodywork (NCTMB), in the exercise of professional accountability will:

*Have a sincere commitment to provide the highest quality of care to those that seek their professional services.

*Represent their qualifications honestly, including education and professional affiliations, and provide only those services which they are qualified to perform.

*Accurately inform clients, other health care practitioners, and the public of the scope and limitations of their discipline.

*Acknowledge the limitations of and contraindications for massage and bodywork and refer clients to appropriate health professionals.

*Provide treatment only where there is reasonable expectation that it will be advantageous to the client.

*Consistently maintain and improve professional knowledge and competence, striving for professional excellence through regular assessment of personal and professional strengths and weaknesses and through continued education training.

*Conduct their business and professional activities with honesty and integrity, and respect the inherent worth of all persons.

*Refuse to unjustly discriminate against clients or other ethical health professionals.

*Safeguard the confidentiality of all client information, unless disclosure is required by law, court order, or absolutely necessary for the protection of the public.

*Respect the client's right to treatment with informed and voluntary consent. The NCTMB practitioner will obtain and record the informed consent of the client, or client's advocate, before providing treatment. This consent may be written or verbal.

*Respect the client's right to refuse, modify, or terminate treatment regardless of prior consent given.

*Provide draping and treatment in a way that ensures the safety, comfort and privacy of the client.

*Exercise the right to refuse to treat any person or part of the body for just and reasonable cause.

*Refrain, under all circumstances, from initiating or engaging in any sexual conduct, sexual activities, or sexualizing behavior involving a client, even if the client attempts to sexualize the relationship.

*Avoid any interest, activity or influence which might be in conflict with the practitioner's obligation to act in the best interests of the client or the profession.

*Respect the client's boundaries with regard to privacy, disclosure, exposure, emotional expression, beliefs, and the client's reasonable expectations of professional behavior. Practitioners will respect the client's autonomy.

*Refuse any gifts or benefits which are intended to influence a referral, decision or treatment that are purely for personal gain and not for the good of the client.

*Follow all policies, procedures, guidelines, regulations, codes, and requirements promulgated by the National Certification Board for Therapeutic Massage and Bodywork.

Code of Ethics

The following is a list of suggested guidelines for appropriate behavior between practitioner and client so that a safe environment is created for both practitioner and client around the issue of sexual boundaries.

1. No sexual contact or intercourse between practitioner and client before, during, or after a treatment session.

2. No sexual contact or dating between practitioner and client during the course of treatment.

3. If the practitioner and client want to have a romantic relationship, the professional relationship must be terminated first.

4. The practitioner is responsible for maintaining appropriate boundaries even if the client is perceived as being seductive.

5. Client undresses and dresses in private.

6. Client has a clear choice as to whether he/she is nude, wears underwear or a smock during treatment.

7. Practitioner never works on or in the genital area or the anus.

8. Practitioner never works on the nipple area of a client.

9. Practitioner uses only the hands, arms, elbows, and feet to massage a client.

10. Practitioner uses only the knee, lateral aspect of the hip and lower leg for bracing.

11. Practitioner never uses the chest, head, face, lips, pelvis or breasts to massage a client.

12. Practitioner does not use inappropriate parts of body for bracing, i.e. front of pelvis, face.

13. Appropriate draping procedures will always be observed.

14. The practitioner refrains from flirting with the clients verbally or otherwise creating a flirtatious atmosphere in the treatment context.

15. The practitioner uses appropriate clinical terminology when speaking about body parts to the client.

16. The practitioner does not make any remarks about the client's body which contain sexual innuendo.

17. The practitioner does not probe intrusively for information about the client's emotional/sexual history, or in any way imply that the client must give such information.

18. If information about the client's emotional/sexual history is communicated, the practitioner does not offer judgments or diagnoses.

19. In cases where the practitioner suspects a sexual abuse history but this is not perceived by the client, the practitioner refrains from imposing his/her opinion on the client.

20. The practitioner must remain within his/her scope of practice and training when dealing with sexual issues. This includes referring to, or working in conjunction with, other practitioners when appropriate for the well-being of the client and the bodyworker.

21. Practitioner seeks informed consent from the client to work on certain parts of the body. For example - high on the thigh, on the chest around breast tissue, buttock, front of the hip near genital area and stomach.

Components of Informed Consent

1. Practitioner gives the client information about the nature of the proposed treatment (body part, type of strokes, pressure, if pain will be felt, etc.) and duration of the treatment.

2. Practitioner gives reasoning/rationale for the proposed treatment.

3. The practitioner and client create and understand a shared objective for the outcome of the treatment.

4. The client feels a sense of free choice with respect to accepting or rejecting the proposed treatment or parts of it, either before or after the treatment begins.

CLIENT FOLDER FORMS

Health History Form

Name _____   Date _____

Address _____   Phone _____

_____   Work phone _____

Sex: M   F   Height _____ Weight _____ Date of birth _____

Contact in case of emergency _____

Reason for wanting massage therapy _____

Have you had massage before? _____ Reason _____

Have you seen a physician in the last two years? _____ Reason _____

_____

Have you had/do you have any of the following conditions?

_____ Allergies   _____ Back injury   _____ Blood clots

_____ Rashes/skin problems _____ Neck injury   _____ Varicose veins

_____ Abdominal pain   _____ Bruises   _____ High blood pressure

_____ Contact lenses   _____ Cancer   _____ Heart disease

_____ Pregnancy   _____ Do you take vitamins? _____ Do you smoke?

_____ Other injury (describe) _____ Surgery in the past year (describe)

_____

Are you taking any drugs or medications? _____   For what condition?

_____

Please list your physician's name and telephone _____

_____

Are there any other medical issues of which we should be aware? _____

_____

   I hereby certify that I have disclosed all information about any condition that may be affected by massage, and I take sole responsiblity for advising the therapist giving the massage as to how it feels, favorably or adversely, and take full responsibility for the results. I understand that all massages will be given by a licensed massage therapist or a student under an instructor's supervision, and I agree that I will hold no party other than myself liable for any treatment or the results thereof.

_____

Client Signature   Date

Personal Information and Financial Agreement

Name _____ Date _____ Home phone _____

Address _____ City _____ Zip code _____

Date of birth _____ Age _____ Marital status   S M W D

No. of children _____ Social security no. _____

Occupation _____ Employer_____

Address _____ Office phone _____

Name of spouse _____ Occupation _____

Employer_____ Office phone _____

Referred by _____ If insurance, name of company _____

Group name _____ Policy no./group no. _____

What is your present complaint? _____ How long? _____

What previous treatment did you seek? _____Were X-rays taken? _____

Is your condition: Improving _____ Getting worse _____ Same _____

Does your condition interfere with: Work _____Sleep_____ Daily routine _____Other _____

Did accident/injury occur at work?_____ Date _____ Time _____

Have you been in an auto accident?   Never____ Past year____ Past 5 yrs. ____Over 5 yrs. ____

Date of auto accident: _____

Describe details of accident: _____
_____
_____

It is understood and agreed that health and accident insurance policies are an arrangement between an insurance carrier and myself._____ will prepare any necessary reports and forms to assist me in making collection from the insurance company and that any amount authorized to be paid directly to _____ will be accredited to my account on receipt. It is further understood that all services rendered me are charged directly to me and that I am personally responsible for payment. I agree to pay for all services at the time they are rendered unless prior arrangements are made.

Patient's Signature _____ Date _____

SOAP Reporting Form

Client _____ Date _____ Student _____

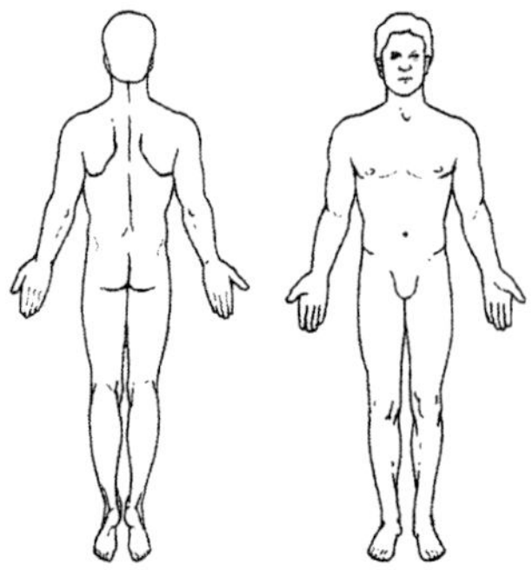

_____

_____

_____

_____

_____

_____

_____

_____

_____

_____

_____

_____

Client _____ Date _____ Student _____

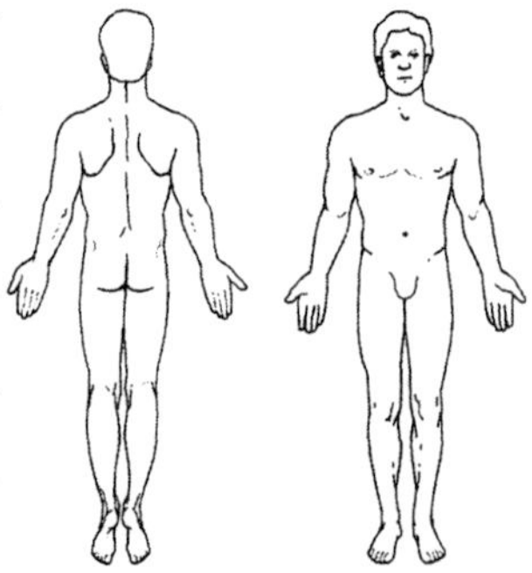

_____

_____

_____

_____

_____

_____

_____

_____

_____

_____

_____

| Pain | (P) | Right | (R) | Depressed, decreased ↓ | Cross fiber friction | XFF | Rotation ↻ |
| Spasm | Sp | Left | (L) | Elevated, increased ↑ | Low back pain | LBP | Tension ten |

Client Financial Record

Case number _____   Patient's name _____

Address _____ Insurance _____ Date _____

Tele. no. _____ Occupation _____ DOB _____ Sex ___ S M W D

Date			Visits and findings	Charges	Paid	Balance
Mo.	Day	Yr.				

**Massage Clinic
Client Information Form**

Name _____ Birth date _____

Address _____ Telephone _____

_____ Business phone _____

City   State   Zip   Social security # _____

Occupation _____ Other activities _____

General health condition _____ Blood pressure _____

Have you any serious chronic illness, operation, chronic virus infections,

or traumatic accidents? _____

Are you in recovery for addictions or abuse? _____

Are you under physician, chiropractor or other health practitioner care? _____

If so, for what condition/s? _____

Are you on any medication? _____ If so, what? _____

Do I have permission to contact your doctor/therapist? _____

Names of physicians, chiropractors or health practitioners: _____

Name _____ Name _____

Address _____ Address _____

Telephone _____ Telephone _____

Why did you come for our services? (relaxation, pain, therapy, etc.) _____

_____

What results would you like to achieve with our work? _____

Have you had any massage therapy before? _____ If so, by whom? _____

How did you find out about our services? _____

Were you referred to this office? _____ By whom? _____

In case of emergency notify: Name _____ Phone _____

I have completed this information form to the best of my knowledge. I understand the massage services are designed to be a health aid and are in no way to take the place of physician care when it is indicated. Information exchanged during any massage session is educational in nature and is intended to help me become more familiar and conscious of my own health status and is to be used at my own discretion. Our time together is precious and I agree to cancel 24 hours in advance. Unless there is an emergency, if I miss an appointment, I agree to pay the full appointment fee.

Date _____ Signature _____

PREGNANCY ROUTINE AND INFANT MASSAGE

▪ PREGNANCY ROUTINE

Positioning. (8 months). Side-lying position.
Pillows:

- One pillow under the baby.
- Two pillows under the top leg.
- One pillow under the head.

Total pillows needed, 7 to 10.

Draping. Normal draping, exposing the body part to be massaged.

Routine

1. Start on posterior back, working up to the shoulder. Concentrate on the low back and hips; these areas take most of the weight of the infant. You may find the sciatic nerve area is painful; work the area under the client's pain threshold.
2. Work across the shoulders in order to balance the body.

3. On the legs, work from the ankle upward to the hip to help drain any excess fluid in the leg. Work the top leg on the lateral side and the lower leg on the medial side in this position.

4. Reposition the client on the other side of the body. Pillow positions will be the same. Repeat steps 1 to 3.

5. Reposition the client supine for a short period of time. Redrape using a breast towel to effect exposure of the abdomen. Position two pillows under the legs; one under the low back; two under the thoracic area; three under the shoulders, neck, and head. (Pillow positions may vary as to the clients' needs.)

6. Work the colon. Clear the left side descending colon first. (Colon will be more lateral than is usual with abdominal massage.) Once the left side is clear, work the entire colon in a clockwise direction. The client should be informed that, in most cases, bowel movement will follow in less than 3 hours.

7. Start preparing the baby by positioning hands crosswise across the baby. Hold hands in touch position for several minutes. Soft effleurage on baby. Rub back and buttocks of baby.

8. Work the legs, arms, and hands of the client as usual.

9. Do the client's neck and face as usual.

If the client is experiencing a lot of hip and low back pain, stretching the leg may help:

- Flex the leg and position the sole of the foot on the medial knee. The therapist's hands stabilize the opposite hip and the flexed knee. Push the flexed knee to the table several times to stretch the adductors. Repeat for the other leg.
- Therapist holds back of the ankle and back of the knee on the flexed leg. As client kicks the leg straight, the therapist pulls the leg to stretch the hip rotators. Keep the leg stabilized at all times. Repeat if necessary. Repeat on the other leg.

▪ INFANT MASSAGE

Massaging the infant after the birth will continue to develop and strengthen the bond between parent and child. Research has shown that babies are healthier, develop better, and are less fussy when regular massage is given. What better way to give your child safe-touch?

General Instructions. Position the baby on parent's outstretched legs or on a bed or floormat. The most important factor is that both child and parent are comfortable and relaxed. Use only light pressure and gentle strokes. Use fingers together or one alone to accomplish the strokes.

Do not massage when the baby has just eaten, has an open cut or inflamed area, has a fever, or is under 4 weeks old. Do include the following strokes in your infant massage.

Water Wheel

1. Paddle across the baby's tummy with the edges of your hands, as if scooping sand.
2. Hold the baby's legs up at the ankles with hand and scoop with the other. Drop baby's legs.
3. Join your thumbs in the middle of his tummy and, with the thumbs flat, push out to the sides.

Sun Moon. With your right palm, shape a half moon from left to right on baby's tummy. Your left palm, meanwhile, circles all the way around, clockwise. As the right hand glides off the skin, the left comes around to complete the circle.

Make a Heart. Palms joined at the center of baby's chest, push out to the shoulders, then move down over the ribs. Glide back up to the chest in a heart-shaped motion. Baby thinks this is great fun. You plant a smooch on his or her tummy and move on in your massage.

SOAP NOTES WITH SIX MASSAGE ROUTINES

▪ SOAP NOTES

- *Subjective assessment.* Information the client gives the therapist before, during, and after the session is included. The client's goals for the session are also included.
- *Objective assessment.* Information the therapist gathers from the interview, health history form, and discussion with the client. The therapist's goals may also be included here. The client's and therapist's goals need to be reconciled.
- *Assessment or application.* What is done during the massage. State modalities used, specific work done, and responses to the work.
- *Plan, procedure, or progress.* Includes plan for the next treatment, what seems to be successful and what does not, self-help homework given the client, and client's reaction to the treatment (Thompson, 1993).

▪ MASSAGE ROUTINE 1—BASIC ROUTINE (USING ALL SEVEN STROKES, FULL BODY)

Position. Client is prone. Use each of the following strokes in the order given: touch, gliding, kneading, friction, vibration, compression, and percussion.

Work each body part three to four times with each stroke before proceeding to the next body part. Proceed from the back to the arm and leg on one side of the body, then to the leg and arm on the other side of the body.

Reposition the client in the supine position. Wherever you left off (for example, right arm posterior), start with the same extremity, anterior position and continue around the body, using all the strokes on each body part.

▪ MASSAGE ROUTINE—SEATED MASSAGE, BASIC ROUTINE

Position. Client is sitting comfortably in massage chair or in a regular chair with the back open to the therapist, or is using a table-topper specially made for massage (see Fig. 9–3). Prop as needed with pillows. Massage is done over regular clothes. Time of treatment should be 10 to 15 minutes. Repeat each move twice. No attempt is made for a return stroke. Therapist stands behind client.

1. Glide hands across shoulders and down back.
2. Press downwards across shoulders using palms of hands. Work medially to laterally in several positions across the shoulders.
3. Press along the spine in the lamina groove, in five to six positions from C7 area to iliac crest, using thurmb or palm of hand.
4. Stabilize one shoulder with one hand and repeat step 3 along the same positions but slightly deeper.
5. Repeat with other hand on other shoulder.
6. Press along quadratis lumborum across the iliac crest in three positions, starting medially 1 inch from spine, and move laterally.
7. Using palm, press and rotate hands across gluteals in three places; working medially to laterally. You may want to kneel to do this more easily.
8. Therapist stands at the side of the client. Support the arm at the wrist with one hand and squeeze the shoulder; deltoids to biceps and triceps.
9. Press down the middle of the arm four or five positions on upper and lower arm.
10. Repeat pressing of arm along radial and ulnar sides of the arm in four or five positions.
11. Squeeze the wrist and spread tissue on the hand, palm downward.
12. Turn palm up and press four or five positions on the arm.
13. Spread the hand, palm up, press base of thumb.
14. Friction each finger between thumb and fingers.
15. Raise the arm to stretch it, vibrate arm, and return it to neutral position.
16. Repeat steps 8 to 15 with the other arm.
17. Press with the thumb along the occiput in four or five positions, working medially to laterally. Repeat on the other side of the head.
18. Knead the neck with one hand, and then the other.
19. Using all fingers, grab the head and gently massage it. (You may want to ask the client first if he or she wants this done.)
20. Re-press the shoulders downwards with both forearms working bilaterally in several positions.
21. Squeeze the upper trapezius muscles, one side at a time.

22. Lift the shoulders up and let them drop naturally.
23. Do a little percussion on the back, using hacking, slapping, or tapping across the shoulders.
24. Feather stroke down the back and arms. Then help the client up out of the chair.

▪ MASSAGE ROUTINE 3—ABDOMEN

This routine should be practiced separately before including it with the full body massage. See Figures E–1 and E–2 for correct hand positioning and direction of strokes in abdominal massage.

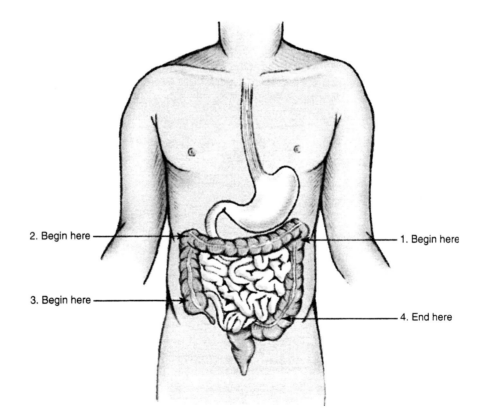

FIGURE E–1. Beginning and ending positions on the colon in abdominal massage.

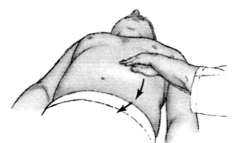

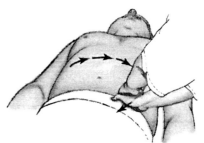

1. Using short strokes massage down descending colon to sigmoid colon.

2. Massage across transverse colon directing short strokes to sigmoid colon.

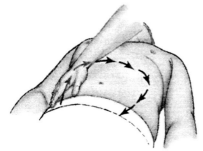

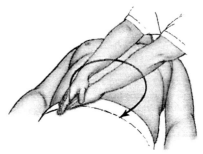

3. Massage up the ascending colon directing short strokes to sigmoid colon.

4. Massage in a circular pattern from ileocecal valve to sigmoid colon. Repeat the four steps again.

FIGURE E–2. Correct hand positioning and direction of strokes in abdominal massage.

Position. Client is supine. The hips and knees are flexed and pillows are added under both for support, allowing the abdomen and the pelvis to relax. Draping should isolate the abdominal area only.

1. Use gliding strokes to the lateral and anterior abdomen. Do the left side to soften the descending colon first. Use short strokes toward the sigmoid colon. Repeat several times before proceeding.
2. Use gliding strokes, working clockwise around the abdomen. You can use alternating hands or one hand only, if you prefer. Use short strokes toward the sigmoid colon first. The direction is up the ascending colon and across the transverse colon.
3. Starting with the ascending colon, perform circular kneading to the abdomen in a clockwise direction.
4. Perform circular friction in a clockwise direction to the abdomen.
5. Repeat steps 1 through 4.

6. Lumbar lift:
   - Slide hands under medial aspect of the rib cage and slide down past the waist to the lumbar region.
   - Place hands on either side of spine.
   - Lift against the lumbar region, vibrating while lifting.
   - Repeat.
7. Return the legs to the table, supporting them as you lift the pillows out.

▪ MASSAGE ROUTINE 4—FULL BODY, INTERMEDIATE ROUTINE

Position. Client is prone.

1. Lubricate and warm the entire back using superficial gliding strokes.
2. Using the palm of the hand, apply circular friction from the iliac crest to the upper trapezius. Work the right side first, then the left side, then both sides simultaneously.
3. Do a figure 8 gliding stroke from hip to shoulders. Use hand over hand for a deeper stroke. Repeat on the other side of the back.
4. Use deep circular friction with the thumbs on either side of the vertebrae, tracing the lamina groove.
5. Knead both sides of the back. Walk around to the other side of the back for comfort and correct body mechanics.
6. Use cross-fiber friction to the rhomboid area, working from the spine towards the scapula.
7. Elevate the shoulder with one hand and work a deep gliding stroke, tracing the edges of the scapula.
8. Repeat steps 6 and 7 for the other side of the back.
9. Move to above the head. Use circular movements around the scapula, upper trapezius, and deltoids.
10. Knead the back of the neck with one hand, then the other.
11. Use deep circular friction with thumbs to the base of the occiput.
12. Work bilateral gliding stroke down the entire back and return the stroke along the sides of the trunk.
13. Avoiding the kidney area (below the 12th rib), do percussion on the back, using hacking, slapping, and tapping.
14. Using the thenar eminence (pad below the thumb), use circular friction over the sacrum and iliac crest area.
15. Vibrate the muscles on either side of the spine.
16. Use deep gliding to the entire back.
17. Feather stroke the entire back.
18. Redrape to cover the back and to uncover the posterior surface of a leg.
19. Apply oil and use superficial strokes over the entire limb.
20. Use circular friction over the bottom of the feet.
21. Squeeze the heel.

22. Use friction to both malleolus bones, using the fingers.
23. Knead the calf.
24. Use deep gliding strokes to the lower leg.
25. Use deep gliding strokes to the thigh.
26. Use circular gliding strokes across the buttocks.
27. Give gliding strokes to the entire limb.
28. Feather stroke from buttocks to feet.
29. Repeat steps 19 to 28 on the other leg.
30. Redrape both legs and uncover same-side arm.
31. Use superficial gliding strokes to cover the entire posterior arm.
32. Knead arm, especially deltoid area.
33. Friction the wrist and elbow.
34. Use gliding strokes to cover the entire arm.
35. Apply light percussion to the entire arm. Use light slapping or tapping only.
36. Feather stroke entire arm.
37. Repeat steps 31 to 36 on the other arm.
38. Redrape and turn the client over.

Position. Supine.

39. Begin with the same arm that you just massaged in the prone position. Uncover the arm.
40. Apply oil and gliding strokes to the full length of the arm.
41. Apply circular friction to each finger and then traction it gently.
42. Knead the palm of the hand.
43. Give deep stroking to the forearm.
44. Flex the elbow and drain the forearm using the C stroke. Work around the limb.
45. Flex arm over the client's shoulder and apply deep gliding strokes, kneading, and friction from elbow to shoulder.
46. Give light traction to the entire arm with vibration. Return arm to table.
47. Feather stroke entire arm.
48. Redrape arm and uncover the same-side leg.
49. Give superficial gliding strokes to the entire leg, ankle to hip.
50. Knead the foot.
51. Friction the top of the foot.
52. Give circular friction to each toe using traction on each toe afterwards.
53. Use knuckles to friction the bottom of the foot.
54. Trace three arches in the foot with the thumbs.
55. Give gliding strokes to the lower legs.
56. Apply circular friction to the sides of the knees, using palms.
57. Trace the patellas with your thumbs.
58. Use gliding strokes on the thighs.
59. Use horizontal strokes on the thighs.
60. Knead the thighs.
61. Feather stroke from hip to foot.

62. Redrape leg and uncover the other leg.
63. Repeat steps 49 to 61 on the other leg.
64. Repeat steps 39 to 47 on the other arm.

Position. Therapist at client's head.

65. Apply oil and begin gliding strokes from the center of the sternum lateral to the anterior deltoid.
66. Reach under shoulder and return medial stroke across the posterior trapezius and under the neck, gliding up to the occipital ridge.
67. Turn head to one side and use short gliding strokes to the lateral neck.
68. Use circular friction to occiput area.
69. Turn head to other side and repeat steps 67 and 68.
70. With heel of hands, use gliding stroke laterally across frontal area of head.
71. Give circular friction to the frontal and temporal area, using thumbs or fingers.
72. Lightly knead ears.
73. Use gliding strokes to the mandible with thumb or fingers.
74. Trace zygomatic arch with fingertips.
75. Rotate head gently.
76. Let client rest before helping up.

▪ MASSAGE ROUTINE 5—SEATED MASSAGE, INTERMEDIATE ROUTINE

Seated massage is often done when clients do not want to position themselves on a massage table or cannot do so. Often, seated massage is done in public places where the removal of clothing is neither wanted nor appropriate. It can be performed on a specially constructed massage chair, on a straight back chair, or using a portable head rest and/or pillows to position the client comfortably.

This routine of legs and feet may be added to a seated chair routine when time allows. Do the upper body as suggested in Routine 2 earlier in the appendix, reserving moves 6 and 7 until the end of the routine. Add this routine after step 24 and start with the 6 and 7 moves. Repeat each move twice.

1. Step 6 from Routine 2. (You may want to kneel to do these.)
2. Step 7 from Routine 2.
3. Place palm over sacrum and friction lightly.
4. Jostle both sides of leg, thigh to ankle, using both hands on the sides of the leg.
5. Press along the quadriceps in three places from the knee to upper thigh, using palm.
6. Knead along the sides of the lower leg, knee to ankle.
7. Friction around the patella in several places, lightly.
8. Trace the ankle bone. (Pick up the leg, supporting the knee, if more convenient.)

9. Do a foot massage, as in reflexology, if possible. Otherwise, proceed using knuckle. Press and twist along the sole of the foot in three lines down the foot.
10. Friction each toe and slightly traction each toe.
11. Trace three arches: two longitudinal, one transverse.
12. Using thumb or knuckle, press all over the bottom of the foot.
13. Squeeze the heel of the foot.
14. Feather stroke down the leg and the foot.
15. Repeat steps 4 to 14 on the other leg.

▪ MASSAGE ROUTINE 6—BASIC SHIATSU ROUTINE

General Rules. Work down the body. Have client turn head frequently to avoid stiff neck. People with low back problems may prefer to keep legs raised, lowering them when they are being worked.

Caution. Avoid varicose veins. Also avoid shiatsu on the abdomen during pregnancy. Avoid heavy pressure on the legs in later stages of pregnancy.

Position. Prone. Work on floor mat.

1. Stretch back to loosen. Apply pressure along side of spine down both sides with palms and then thumbs.
2. Press along sacrum, squeeze the sides of buttocks and use elbow on the upper curve.
3. Press down center of each leg, with palm and then knees. Press ankle points and stretch legs. Press down both sides of legs. Walk on each sole of foot.
4. Press along top of each shoulder. Rotate scapulas. Press along spine between shoulder blades. Loosen shoulder muscles with feet.

Position. Supine.

5. Lean on front of shoulders to open the client's energy. Press along spaces between ribs to relieve congestion. Do neck meridians and circle sides of neck. Stretch the neck.
6. Run your fingers through the hair and gently pull it. Massage ears. Do points on face, eyes, temple, jaw, nostrils, and mouth as well as along midline of head.
7. Treat the inner surface of the arm, palm up, then palm downward. Pull fingers and point between thumb and forefinger. Shake arm to loosen and relax it. Repeat on the other arm.
8. Work clockwise around hara (abdomen). Gently press undersides of ribs, and down midline to navel. Rock the torso.
9. Press down inside of each leg, then front of thigh. Rotate kneecap and press point just below the knee. Press down inside skin. Stretch foot and repeat on other leg.

RESOURCE AND INFORMATION LIST

Academy for Myotherapy and
   Physical Fitness
9 School Street
Lenox, MA 01240

Acupressure Institute
15333 Shattush Avenue
Berkeley, CA 94709

American International Reiki
   Association
2210 Wilshire Boulevard,
   Suite 831
Santa Monica, CA 90405

American Massage Therapy
   Association (AMTA)
Department of Information
820 Davis Street
Suite 100
Evanston, IL 60201

Massage Therapy Journal
820 Davis Street
Suite 100
Evanston, IL 60201

American Polarity Therapy Association
2888 Bluff Street, No. 149
Boulder, CO 80310

American Shiatsu Association
295 Huntington Avenue
Room 205
Boston, MA 02015

Amma Institute
1596 Post Street
San Fransisco, CA 94109

Aroma Vera (aromatherapy)
Box 3609 R
Culver City, CA 90231

Associated Bodywork and Massage
  Professionals
28677 Buffalo Park Road
Evergreen, CO 80439–7347

Associated Professional Massage
  Therapists and Allied Health
  Practitioners International
1746 Cole Blvd.
Golden, CO 80401

Aveda (aromatherapy)
321 Lincoln Street, NE
Minneapolis, MN 55413

Body Support Systems
PO Box 337
300 E. Hersey
Ashland, OR 97520

Bonnie Prudden, Inc.
Myotherapy School
7800 East Speedway
Tucson, AZ 85710

Brennan, Barbara (energy healing)
School of Healing
PO Box 2005
East Hampton, NY 11987

Barnes, John (myofascial therapy)
105 Leopard Road, Suite One
Paoli, PA 19301

Chaitow, Leon, DO
26 Dene Close
Willingborough, Northamptonshire
United Kingdom NN8 3QP

Colorado Cranial Institute
466 Maine Street
Boulder, CO 80302

Colorcrafts (color therapy)
1010 Sand Branch Road
Black Mountain, NC 28711

Doctor Wilkinson's Hot Springs
  (mud baths)
1507 Lincoln Avenue
Calistoga, CA 94515

Eisenberg, Michael (Thai massage)
1539 Peace Lane
Bow, WA 98232

Equissage
PO Box 447
Round Hill, VA 22141

Farnell, Stuart (equine therapies)
PO Box 33676
Palm Beach Gardens, FL 33420

Heller, Joseph (Hellerwork)
c/o Body of Knowledge
415 N. Mt. Shasta Boulevard, no. 4
Mt. Shasta, CA 96067

International Association of Infant
  Massage Instructors
PO Box 10103
Portland, OR 97216

International Association of Pfrimmer
  (deep muscle therapists)
PO Box 807
Smithfield, NC 27577

International Institute of Reflexology
PO Box 12642
St. Petersburg, FL 35733

International Massage Association
3000 Connecticut Avenue, NW, Suite 308
Washington, DC 20008

Kushi Institute (do-in)
PO Box 1100
Brookline, MA 02147

Myotherapy Institute Research Center
3350 South 2300 East
Salt Lake City, UT 84109

National Certification Board for
   Therapeutic Massage and Bodywork
   (NCBTMB)
National Certification Exam
8201 Greensboro Drive, Suite 300
McLean, VA 22102

National sports massage certification
   and sports team information
   (*see American Massage Therapy
   Association*)

Neuromuscular Integration and
   Structural Alignment (NISA)
c/o Jean Loving
SNI School of Massage (Seminar
   Network International)
518 North Federal Highway
Lake Worth, FL 33460

North American Vodder Association
   of Lymphatic Therapy
PO Box 861
Chesterfield, OH 44026

Ohashi Institute (shiatsu)
12 West 27th Street
New York, NY 10001

On Site Massage Association
   (chair massage)
1596 Post Street
San Fransisco, CA 94109

Osmosis (enzyme baths)
PO Box 1713
Sebastopol, CA 96473

Palmer, David (chair or seated
   massage)
584 Costia Street, No. 555
San Francisco, CA 94114

The Rolf Institute
PO Box 1868
Boulder, CO 80306

Shaw Myotherapy Institute
6417 Loisdale Road, Suite 309
Springfield, VA 22150

Shea Educational Group, Inc.
Michael Shea
13875 Oleander Avenue
Juno Beach, FL 33408

Spa Finders Guide—Spa Finders'
   Travel Arrangements, Ltd.
784 Broadway
New York, NY 10003-4856

St. John Neuromuscular
Paul St. John
11211 Prosperity Farms Road, D-325
Palm Beach Gardens,
   FL 33410-3487

TEAM News International
   (equine massage)
Box 5 Site 9
RR 8
Edmonton, Alberta
Canada T5L 4H5

Therapeutic Touch (Dolores Krieger)
c/o Nurse Healers and Professional
   Associates Cooperative, Inc.
175 Fifth Avenue, Suite 3399
New York, NY 10010

Touch for Health Enterprises Store
1200 North Lake Avenue
Pasadena, CA 91104

Touch For Health Foundation
1174 North Lake Avenue
Pasadena, CA 91104

Touch Research Institute (TRI)
University of Miami Medical School
Dominion Tower
1400 NW 10th, 6th floor
Miami, FL 33136

Trager Institute
10 Mill Street
Mill Valley, CA 94941

Upledger Institute (cranial–sacral
   therapies and clinic)
11211 Prosperity Farms Road
Palm Beach Gardens, FL 33410

Van Why, Richard (bodywork
   knowledge base and research)
123 East Eighth Street
Suite 121
Frederick, MD 21701

World Research Foundation
   (color therapy)
15300 Ventura Boulevard,
   Suite 405
Sherman Oaks, CA 91403

The Zero Balancing Association
Fritz Smith
PO Box 1727
Capitola, CA 95010

BIBLIOGRAPHY

Amber, Reuben: *Color Therapy.* New York, Aurora Press, 1983.

Balsdon, JPVD: *Life and Leisure in Ancient Rome.* London, Bodley Head Ltd., 1969.

Beck, Mark F: *Theory and Practice of Therapeutic Massage,* 2nd ed. New York, Delmar Publishers, 1994.

Benjamin, Ben: "Guidelines for Safe and Ethical Contact." *Massage Therapy Journal,* winter 1992a.

Benjamin, Ben: "Sexual Misconduct: An Informational Brochure for Consumers of Health Care Services." *Massage Therapy Journal,* summer 1992b.

Benjamin, Ben: "Understanding Boundary Violations in Therapist–Client Relationship." *Massage Therapy Journal,* fall 1991.

Benjamin, Ben: "Sexual Abuse Within the Health Care Field." *Massage Therapy Journal,* spring 1990.

Benjamin, Ben, and Chello, Daphne: "Dual Roles and Other Ethical Considerations." *Massage Therapy Journal,* spring 1992.

Brennan, Barbara A: *Hands of Light A Guide to Healing Through the Human Energy Field.* New York, Bantam Books, 1987.

Casaopiro, Jerome: *Daily Life in Ancient Rome.* New Haven, Yale University Press, 1968.

Chaitow, Leon: *Modern Neuromuscular Technique.* New York, Churchill, Livingstone, 1996a.

Chaitow, Leon: *Muscle Energy Techniques.* New York, Churchill Livingstone, 1996b.

Chaitow, Leon: *Positional Release Techniques.* New York, Churchill Livingstone, 1996c.

Chaitow, Leon: *Soft Tissue Manipulation.* Rochester, VT, Healing Arts Press, 1988.

Cohen, Don: *An Introduction to Craniosacral Theory, Anatomy, Function and Treatment.* Berkeley, CA, North Atlantic Books, 1995.

Covey, Stephen R: *The Seven Habits of Highly Effective People: Powerful Lessons in Personal Change.* New York, Simon & Schuster, 1989.

Covey, Stephen R, Merrill, Roger A, and Merrill, Rebecca R: *First Things First.* New York, Simon & Schuster, 1994.

Culpepper, Nicholas: *Culpepper's Complete Herbal.* London, Foulsham.

Cyriax, James: *Textbook of Orthopedic Medicine.* London, Bailliere Tindall, 1984.

DeDomenico, Giovanni, and Wood, Elizabeth: *Beard's Massage,* 4th ed. Philadelphia, Saunders, 1997.

Dinshah, Darius: *Let There Be Light.* Malaga, NJ, Dinshah Health Society, 1995.

Feltman, John, ed: *Hands-on Healing: Massage Remedies for Hundreds of Health Problems.* Emmaus, PA, Rodale Press, 1989.

Field, Tiffany: *Current Research Report.* Miami, Touch Institute, 1997.

Fitzhenry, Robert, ed: *The Harper Book of Quotations,* 3rd ed. New York, Harper, 1993.

Flexner Stuart, ed: *Random House Dictionary of the English Language.* New York, Random House, 1987.

Fritz, Sandy: *Fundamentals of Therapeutic Massage.* St. Louis, Mosby, 1995.

Goleman, Daniel, and Gourin, Joel, eds: *Mind–Body Medicine: How to Use Your Mind for Better Health.* Yonkers, NY, Consumer Reports Books, 1993.

Grant, Michael: *Gladiators.* New York, Delacort Press, 1968.

Halpern, Steven: *Sound Health.* New York, Harper & Row, 1985.

Hoppenfeld, Stanley: *Physical Examination of the Spine & Extremities.* New York, Appleton-Century-Crofts, 1976.

Jones, Lawrence: *Strain & Counterstrain.* Colorado Springs, CO, American Academy of Osteopathy, 1981.

Kellogg, John Harvey: *The Art of Massage.* Self-published, 1895.

King, Robert: *Performance Massage.* Champaign, IL, Human Kinetics, 1993.

Knapp, Joan E, and Antonusic, Eileen J: *A National Study of the Profession of Massage Therapy and Bodywork.* Princeton, Knapp & Associates, 1990.

Kunz, K and Kunz, B: *The Complete Guide to Foot Reflexology.* Englewood Cliffs, NJ, Prentice Hall, 1982.

La Fleur, Myrna Weber, and Starr, Winifred K: *Exploring Medical Language: A Student-Directed Approach.* St. Louis, Mosby, 1994.

Lowe, Whitney: *Functional Assessment in Massage Therapy.* Yachets, OR, Pacific Orthopedic Massage, 1995.

Lowen, A: *Bioenergetics.* New York, Penguin, 1975.

MacKendrick, Paul, et al., eds: *Greece and Rome: Builders of our World.* Washington, DC, National Geographic Society, 1968.

Mattes, Aaron F: *Active Isolated Stretching.* Self-published, 1995.

Memmler, Ruth L, and Wood, Dena Lin: *The Human Body in Health and Disease.* 5th ed. Philadelphia, Lippincott, 1983.

Moor, Fred B, Peterson, Stella, Manwell, Ethel, Noble, Mary, and Muench, Gertrude. *Manual of Hydrotherapy and Massage.* Oshawa, Ontario, Pacific Press, 1964.

Moore, Gloria: *Isolate and Stretch Effectively.* Self-published. Ft. Pierce, FL, 1995.

Moyers, Bill: *Healing and the Mind.* New York, Doubleday, 1993.

Mulvihill, Mary Lou: *Human Diseases: A Systematic Approach,* 2nd ed. Stamford, CT, Appleton & Lange, 1987.

O'Rourke, Maureen: *Natural Healing With Water, Herbs and Sunlight.* Miami, Educating Hands, 1995.

Paoli, Ugo Enrico: *Rome: Its People, Life, and Customs.* Essex, England, Longman, 1967.

Phinney, E, ed: *Cambridge Latin Course: Unit 1.* Cambridge, Cambridge University Press, 1988.

Rattray, Fione: *Massage Theory: An Approach to Treatments.* Toronto, Ontario, Massage Therapy Texts and MA Versch Consultants, 1994.

Reich, W: *Character Analysis.* New York, Simon & Schuster, 1972.

Rolf, Ida: *Rolfing: The Integration of Human Structures.* New York, Harper & Row, 1977.

Rouse, WHD, translator: Homer, *The Odyssey.* New York, Penguin, 1937.

Schultz, R. Louis, and Feitis, Rosemary: *The Endless Web.* Berkeley, CA, North Atlantic Books, 1996.

Seldes, George: *The Great Quotations.* New York, Carol, 1993.

Selye, Hans: *The Stress of Life,* 2nd ed. New York, McGraw-Hill, 1978.

Selye, Hans: *Stress Without Distress.* New York, Lippincott Co, 1974.

Shea, Michael: *The Myofascial Release Textbook.* Juno Beach, FL, Shea Educational Group, 1995.

Shen, Peijian: *Massage for Pain Relief: A Step by Step Guide.* New York, Random House, 1996.

Siegel, Bernie S: *How to Live Between Office Visits.* New York, Harper Collins, 1993.

Siegel, Bernie S: *Peace, Love and Healing.* New York, Harper & Row, 1989.

Sohn, Tina, and Finando, Donna: *Amma: The Ancient Art of Oriental Healing.* Rochester, VT, Healing Arts Press, 1988.

Stillerman, Elaine: *The Encyclopedia of Bodywork.* New York, Facts on File, 1996.

Tappan, Frances M: *Healing Massage Technique: Classic, Holistic, and Emerging Methods.* Stamford, CT, Appleton Lange, 1998.

Taylor, Kyles: *The Ethics of Caring.* Santa Cruz, CA, Hansford Mead, 1995.

Thibodeau, Gary A, and Patton, Kevin P: *The Human Body in Health and Disease.* St. Louis, Mosby Year Book, 1992.

Thie, John: *Touch for Health.* Marina del Rey, CA, De Vorss, 1973.

Thomas, Clayton, ed: *Taber's Cyclopedic Medical Dictionary,* 15th ed. Philadelphia, Davis, 1981.

Thompson, A, Skinnir, A, and Priecy, J: *Tidy's Physiotherapy,* 12th ed. Oxford, Butterworth & Heinmann, 1990.

Thompson, Diana: *Hands Heal: Documentation for Massage Therapists. A Guide to SOAP Charting.* Self-published, 1993.

Travell, Janet, and Simons, David G: *Myofascial Pain and Dysfunction: The Trigger Point Manual.* Baltimore, Williams & Wilkins, 1983.

Upledger, John, and Vrederriydm, F: *Craniosacral Therapy.* Seattle, Eastland Press, 1983.

Upledger, John: *Craniosacral Therapy II: Beyond the Dura.* Seattle, Eastland Press, 1987.

Van Why, Richard: *The Bodywork Knowledge Base: Lectures on the History of Massage.* New York, Self-published, 1991.

West, Ovida M: *The Magic of Massage—A New and Holistic Approach.* Mamaroneck, NY, Hastings House, 1990.

Wood, Elizabeth, and Becker, Paul: *Beard's Massage,* 3rd ed. Philadelphia, Saunders, 1981.

Worwood, Valerie Ann: *The Fragrant Mind.* Novato, CA, New World Library, 1996.

Yates, John A: *A Physician's Guide to Therapeutic Massage.* Vancouver, Massage Therapists Association of British Columbia, 1990.

Yates, John A: *Physiological Effects of Therapeutic Massage and Their Application to Treatment.* Vancouver, Massage Therapists Association of British Columbia, 1990.

GLOSSARY

A

Acupressure: Therapy based on relieving trigger points associated with meridian lines.

Acupuncture: Ancient Oriental therapy that uses special needles inserted along meridian lines.

Adhesion: A fibrous band holding parts together.

Aesculapius: Ancient Greek god of healing.

Affusion: Hydrotherapy technique of washes.

Allied health field: Any technical field supporting modern medical practice, including many bodywork therapies and associated therapies.

Amma: Ancient healing system that uses the Oriental theories of energy channels or meridians in bodywork. Deep pressure and point manipulation are two techniques employed.

Anatomy: The study of the gross structure of the body.

Antiseptic: An agent that disinfects.

Aromatherapy: The use of scents as in essential oils to aid the healing processs.

Aseptic: A sterile condition free from germs.

Assessment: The third component of SOAP notes. The evaluation of a client's condition to be used to decide on an appropriate treatment plan.

Autoclave: A dry heat cabinet used to sanitize objects used in treatment.

Ayurvedic medicine: An ancient Indian medicine based on the ritual of using oil to anoint.

B

Bacilla: A type of bacteria causing tuberculosis, diphtheria, typhoid fever, etc.

Bacteria: Unicellular organisms having both plant and animal characteristics; also called germs or microbes.

Bell's palsy: A neurological disease that affects the facial nerves, usually unilaterally.

Bindegewebsmassage: A type of massage developed by Elizabeth Dicke, based on the belief that organic disturbances follow vascular channels over arterial reflexes.

Body–mind: A way of thinking that links the body and mind as one unit.

Body reading: A form of body assessment that uses visual clues to evaluate a client's thoughts, feelings, behavior, and past experiences.

Bodywork: A term that encompasses many hands-on theories.

Boundary: An invisible line or professional limit that separates the therapist and the client.

Burnout: A term used to depict a state of extreme fatigue and stress at which point a person can no longer carry on his or her regular work.

Bursitis: An inflammation of the bursa capsule, as in the shoulder or knee.

C

Carpal tunnel syndrome: A pathology involving the carpal tunnel of the wrist in which weakness, numbness, and pain develop from repetitive motion.

Certification: A document awarded for achieving some kind of standard of education. This can include completing a course of study or for passing an examination (e.g., National Certification Exam).

Chakras: The energy centers along the trunk of the body, each of which is associated with a major organ.

Chi (qi, ki): The energy flow through the body as described by ancient cultures.

Chinese traditional medicine: A branch of modern Chinese medicine that includes exercise, acupuncture, massage, and the use of herbs in the healing process.

Client consent: Verbal or written agreement by the client to proceed with the treatment plan as discussed with the therapist.

Cocci: A form of bacteria which causes abscesses, blood poisoning, and pneumonia.

Code of ethics: A set of professional rules and regulations agreed to by the members of a particular professional group.

COMTAA: Commission on Massage Training Accreditation/Approval. An independent board set up by the American Massage Therapy Association (AMTA) to establish and enforce standards in the massage profession and in schools of massage for the purpose of educating and accrediting individuals.

Compression: The art of compressing tissue of the body as in the massage compression stroke.

Confidentiality: A condition or state where the therapist does not release client information unless client permission is granted.

Connective tissue: One of the tissues of the body that connects and supports the organs and other structures of the body.

Consultation: The meeting between the client and therapist to obtain information concerning a client's health.

Contraindication: Pathological condition for which massage is not indicated, either because it would be harmful or wouldn't help the condition.

Contusion: A bruise or injury, usually from a blow.

Cranial–sacral technique: A bodywork system developed by Dr. John Upledger that manipulates the cranial and sacral fluid system of the body as well as the bones of the skull.

Cross-directional stretching: A manipulation that pulls the muscle fibers against the fiber direction and does not require joint movement.

Cryotherapy: The use of ice in therapy.

Cupping: A massage percussion stroke used on the back and chest of the client to loosen congestion in the lungs and pleural cavities.

Cycle of dependence: A term used to describe the dependence of a client on a professional healthcare giver to keep them healthy and well.

D

Diagnosis: The identification of a diseased condition by its symptoms and history.

Diaphragmatic breathing: Breathing deeply so as to affect the diaphragm of the body.

Diploma: An award given in recognition of completion of a body of knowledge.

Directions: A category of medical terms used to locate positions on the human body.

Disclosure: The therapist informs the client of the treatment plan.

Disease crisis: An emergency in a disease that signals medical intervention.

Disinfectant: A chemical product known to destroy the germs of disease.

Draping procedure: The process used to drape a client for massage, to assure safety and modesty.

E

Edema: Swelling of tissue due to fluid retention.

Endangerment site: Specific area of the body that may be dangerous when massaged, usually due to the presence of underlying vessels and/or nerves.

Endorphin: Naturally occurring chemical with analgesic properties; may be released in the brain when massage is given.

Energetic approach and/or model: Bodywork that deals with the energies of the body.

Equine massage: Massage given to horses.

Exudate: Accumulation of fluid in a cavity.

F

Fasciae: The layers of connective tissue membrane that surround organs and other structures in the body.

Felony: A major crime.

Fibromyalgia or fibrocystic syndrome: A pathological condition of inflammation of the white fibrous connective tissue in the body.

Fight-or-flight response: The body's initial reaction to perceived stress.

Fission: The act of breaking or splitting apart.

Fomite: Any substance that adheres to and transmits infectious material.

Friction: A massage stroke which compresses and lifts the tissue.

Fulling: A compression stroke in massage that broadens the tissue.

Fumigant: Chemicals used to disinfect a room.

Fungi: Plant-like organisms, single-celled, like yeast filaments as in molds.

G

Gait: A person's manner of walking.

Geriatric massage: Massage for the elderly population.

Gliding: A superficial massage stroke using long sliding strokes using a variety of pressures.

Golgi tendons: Organ in the muscles with sensory receptors detecting changes in the muscles and bones.

Ground substance: The matrix or base material of fascia in the body.

H

Healing crisis: A detoxifying phase of the healing process.

Hemispheres of the brain: Left and right sections of the brain, each with its own specific tasks to perform.

Hippocrates: An ancient Greek physician (460–377 BC) considered to be the father of medicine and the originator of the Hippocratic oath taken by physicians today.

Homeostasis: State of balance between the inside of the body and the environment outside.

HOPS: An assessment tool including the client's history, observation, palpation by the therapist, and special orthopedic tests if needed.

Hydrotherapy: Use of water in its three forms—liquid, solid, or vapor—in the treatment of the body.

I

Indication: When specific medical conditions are present, a massage modality is advised to alleviate or help the condition.

Inflammation: Presence of an inflamed state in the body. Characterized by swelling, pain, redness, and heat.

Informed consent: Process of informing the client of aspects of treatments to be performed and receiving permission to perform them from the client.

Ischemia: Heat and redness on the skin due to constricted blood flow in the muscles.

Isokinetic contraction: Muscle contraction in which the client moves the joint through its range-of-motion and the therapist uses partial resistance.

Isometric contraction: Muscle contraction in which the ends of the muscle or body part affected do not move.

Isotonic contraction: Muscle contraction in which the tissue between the ends of the muscle does change.

J

Jin shin do: A bodywork technique that uses deep finger pressure on acupoints to release tension and stress in the muscles.

Joint movement: Movement made by the joints, often called range-of-motion in massage.

K

Ki (qi, chi): The energy flow through the body as described by ancient cultures.

Kneading: A massage stroke that lifts, squeezes, and rolls the tissue.

L

License: A document issued by the state or regulating agency as a requirement for business or practicing a profession.

Longitudinal stretching: Stretching of muscles in the direction of the fibers to lengthen them.

Lymphatic drainage or massage: A bodywork method that aids the lymphatic system of the body to cleanse itself.

Lymphocyte: A white blood cell that has less protoplasma than a monocyte.

M

Mainstream medical approach: The theory and practice of clinical massage directed towards the medical field, such as in hospitals and medical clinics.

Manual lymph drainage: Another name for lymphatic drainage bodywork developed by Dr. Emil Vodder.

Massage: The art and science of treating the body with hands-on work. The application of various hands-on strokes, such as friction and kneading, to the muscles of the body.

Medical massage approach (see mainstream medical approach): A system of clinical massage used in the medical field, such as in hospitals and medical clinics.

Meridian or meridian line: Channel of energy running through the body and connected to various organs.

Metazoans: Member of the primary division of animal kingdom having an outer and inner wall; higher than protozoan.

Microorganism: Microscopic organism such as bacteria, fungi, and viruses.

Mind–body: The complex connections between various components of the human body and mind.

Monocyte: A large leukocyte having more protoplasma than a lymphocyte.

Moxibustion: Ancient Chinese method of cleansing the body by lighting the herb mori (mugwort) and placing it on the skin to reduce inflammation.

Muscle testing: A method of using muscle movement and strength to test various body parts and various objects.

Myofascial pain: Pain caused by hardening or sticking of fascia and muscles.

Myofascial technique: Massage method used to treat the fascia and muscles of the body by stretching, softening, and spreading the connective tissue.

N

Necrosis: An area in the muscle or bone tissue that has died, surrounded by healthy tissue.

Neuromuscular therapy: Soft tissue therapy aimed at the nervous system and the muscular system.

Neuromuscular Integration and Structural Alignment (NISA): A method of bodywork that realigns the body by working on soft tissue.

Nociceptor: Nerve cell that senses pain.

O

Objective assessment: The gathering of measurable information from a client to be used in the development of a treatment plan.

Oriental massage model: A variety of modalities based on Oriental principles of meridians, chi energy, etc.

Orthobionomy: A type of bodywork based on the body's self-correcting reflexes. Passive positioning methods are used as well as mental/emotional releases, which reduce muscular tension.

Osteoporosis: Softening and thinning of bones that may lead to fractures.

P

Pain–spasm–pain cycle: A vicious circle of pain, steady contraction of muscles and stimulated pain receptors, spasms, and more pain.

Pain threshold: The point at which pain is felt, on a scale from 1 to 10.

Palpation: Assessment of the body through touch.

Parasite: An organism that lives within, on, or at the expense of another organism.

Paresthesia: Sensation of numbness, prickling, or tingling.

Pathogen: A microorganism or substance capable of producing a disease.

Percussion: A massage stroke; the striking of a series of rapid blows to the body to stimulate it.

Phantom pain: The pain felt by persons after an amputation of a limb.

Physiology: The study of the functions of the body.

Piezoelectric current: A small electric current, produced by compression and similar to that found in crystals, which runs in the spaces between fascial layers. When maintained, the tissue stays soft. When reduced by trauma, the tissue hardens.

Plan, procedure, or progress: The fourth component of SOAP notes which includes the plan for the next treatment and the client's reaction to treatment and homework treatment.

Plantar fascitis: Inflammation of the connective tissue investing the tendons on the sole of the foot.

Postural assessment: See body reading.

Practitioner: Person who practices a discipline (e.g., person doing massage).

Pressure point: Specific point along the meridians that can become painful when congestion or imbalance is present.

Professional boundary: The border or line between a client and the professional.

Professional demeanor: The professional way a practitioner behaves, including their language and appearance.

Proprioception: In body tissue, the body's awareness of position, posture, movement, and changes in equilibrium.

Protozoa: The simplest animals, mostly unicellular.

Psychoneuroimmunology: A new body of knowledge and study that combines the mind, nerves, and immune system of the body.

Pulsed muscle energy procedure: A procedure that engages the barrier of the muscle movement by using resistive constrictions to introduce mechanical pumping of the muscle.

Q

Qi (chi, ki): The energy flow through the body as described by ancient cultures.

R

Range-of-motion (ROM): The actions of a joint as it moves through all of its movements.

Reciprocal inhibition: A technique of bodywork which relaxes a target muscle as the tone increases in its antagonist.

Referral: The process of sending a client to another professional for specific diagnosis or treatment.

RICE: *R*est, *i*ce, *c*ompression, and *e*levation.

Rickettsiae: Microorganisms parasitic in ticks and lice and transmissable to animals and man (e.g., typhus).

Right of refusal: The client's right to stop the treatment or to refuse it at any time.

Role-playing: An educational method that aids learning and understanding by temporarily taking on the characterization and behavior of another person.

Rolfing®: A type of bodywork that aligns body parts by manipulating the connective tissue, founded by Dr. Ida Rolf.

S

Safe touch: Touch performed in such a way that the client experiences no harm or fear.

Sciatic nerve lesion: Altered tissue of the sciatic nerve areas across the posterior pelvis and down the posterior thigh due to inflammation of that nerve.

Scope of practice: The intentions and professionally accepted methods used by practitioners in a profession.

Sexual impropriety: Any behavior, comment, expression or gesture that is seductive, sexual in nature, or demeaning to the client.

Shaman: An ancient word for healer/priest.

Skin rolling: A kneading technique in massage that lifts and rolls the tissue.

SOAP notes: (SOAP stands for Subjective assessment, Objective assessment, Assessment or application, and Plan, procedure, or progress.) Treatment notes derived from client and therapist interaction.

"Spill" of body fluids: The release of body fluids from a client onto massage linens.

Spindle cell: Type of proprioceptor in the muscle.

Spirilla: A type of bacteria which causes syphilis.

Staphylocci: Bacteria that cause inflammation on the skin.

Strain–counterstrain technique (or positional release): A method used to reset the neuromuscular mechanisms in a muscle by positioning a body part.

Streptococci: A type of bacteria that causes blood poisoning.

Stress: A physical, mental, or emotional response to conditions in the environment and everyday life.

Stretching and lengthening: A mechanical means of pulling tissue to increase mobility and reduce stress. Pulling the tissue in the direction of the fibers helps to reset the stretch reflex mechanism in the muscle's spindle cells and Golgi tendon organs near the musculotendinous junctions.

Structural alignment: A type of bodywork that focuses on the connective tissue to change posture and biomechanisms in the body.

Subjective assessment: First component in SOAP notes method; includes what the client says and their behavior.

Suppuration: The formation of pus.

Swedish massage: A Western massage system based on five strokes and named for the place it originated.

Systemic condition: Any physiological condition that affects the whole body.

T

Tai chi: A holistic system of exercise based on balancing the flow of energy in the body and mind.

Tension: The result of coping with stressors of everyday life. Symptoms include backaches, headaches, grinding the teeth, and TMJ.

Thalassotherapy: The use of salt water in a hydrotherapy program.

Therapeutic massage: Massage performed with the aim to provide treatment for a specific conditon.

Therapeutic touch: An energy method of bodywork developed by Dolores Krieger that works above the body.

Touch or touching stroke: The art of touching a person in a nonthreatening way such as a handshake or in palpation, used as the first stroke in massage.

Trager®: A type of bodywork that uses rocking of the body in order to affect the joints, connective tissue, and nervous systems of the body.

Treatment plan: An outline procedure developed by the therapist and agreed to by the client for therapy, based on information gathered from a health history form, questioning and discussion with the client, and palpation.

Trigger point: Hyperirritable spot on the body that elicits pain when compressed. Normal tissue is not painful.

Tsubos: Pressure points based on acupuncture points as in shiatsu.

V

Vector: A directional line of force or energy in the body.

Vibrational therapy or energy therapy: Type of bodywork that uses vibration and energy as part of therapy.

Vibration stroke: A Swedish massage stroke that includes oscillating, quivering, or trembling of tissues, performed quickly and repeatedly.

Virus: A parasitic pathogenic agent that transmits disease. It may cause the common cold, smallpox, measles, mumps, etc.

W

Watsu: A form of underwater shiatsu, similar to rebirthing.

Wellness: The state of feeling well in body, mind, and emotions or spirit. This state is far above just feeling no pain; it is an integration of all parts of a human being.

Whiplash: Injury to the cervical spine and connective tissue surrounding it, usually caused by the sudden jerking forward and backward of the neck, as in an auto accident.

XYZ

Yin and yang: The Oriental belief that items and body parts can be classified as opposing forces; balance is the key.

Yoga: A form of exercise that combines concentration, muscular control, breathing, and relaxation in performing body postures and positions.

Zero balancing: A type of bodywork based on the energetic model developed by Dr. Fritz Smith.

Zone therapy: Another name for reflexology, based on the 10 zones of the body and the reflex ability of the body.

INDEX

Abdominal massage
  in pregnancy, 240–41
Abuse cases, 65–66
Accident prevention, 50
Aching pain, 27, 213–14
Acupoints, 151
Acupressure, 116, 151, 154
Acupuncture, 151, 154
Acute inflammation, 212–13
Acute pain, 213
Addiction
  massage for, 244
Adhesions, 212
Aesculapius, 3
Affusions, 217
AIDS patients, 38
Algae, 44
Alpinus, Prospero, 4
American Association of Masseurs and Masseuses, 7
American Massage Therapy Association (AMTA),
    7, 8, 16, 242
  Code of Ethics, 17–18
Amma (Amna), 57, 151
Anatomy, 54
Anderson, Ron, 56
Animal massage, 165, 167–70
Ankles, 230
Antagonistic contraction, 132
Antiseptics, 44
Arms
  care of, 200, 204–206

positions of, 61
  self-stretching exercises, 204
Aromatherapy, 116, 165, 166–67
Art of Massage, The (Kellogg), 6
Aseptic techniques, 47
Assessment, 173–183
  defined, 174
  HOPS tool, 175–76
  muscle testing, 176–78
  quick tools, 178–80
  referrals, 176
  SOAP notes, 174–175
Athletes
  massage for, 10, 241–42, 246
Athletic teams, 10
Aura balancing, 160
Aura stroking, 96
Autoclave, 45
Averros, 4
Avicenna, 4

Bacilli, 45, 46
Back
  low, self-stretching exercises, 192–94
  self-stretching exercises, 200, 202–203
Bacteria, 45
Balance, 188
Ballistic stretching, 114, 192
Baths, 217, 223

Beard, Gertrude, 8
Beard's Massage (Beard), 8
Beating, 107
Bell's palsy, 229–30, 245
Benjamin, Ben, 70
Biases
of massage therapists, 17–19
Bicipital tendinitis test, 239
Bilos, 146
Bindegewebsmassage, 7, 11, 128
Bio-energetics, 7
Body reading, 59–66, 190
Bodywork, 14, 57
Bodywork Knowledge Base (Van Why), 59
Body wraps, 217
Boundaries, 19, 61
Bowen technique, 128, 129
Breathing
deep breathing exercises, 190, 191
during exercise, 192
pattern, 61
techniques, 117
Burning pain, 27, 213–14
Burnout, 187–88
self-care tips, 188
Burns
cold water therapy for, 221
Bursitis, 227–229
Buttocks, 246

Caesar, Julius, 4
Camus, Albert, 13
Cancer, 245–46
Carpal tunnel syndrome, 235–38, 238
Case studies, 37, 123–24, 180–83, 244–47, 249–50
Celsus, Dr. Aulus, 4
Certification, 8–9, 16–17
Chair massage, 10. *See* Seated massage
Chairs
for seated massage, 159
Chaitow, Boris, 139
Chaitow, Leon, 144
Chakras, 160
Channels, 149–52
Chi (qi, ki), 10, 57, 149
Chill-and-stretch technique, 117, 118, 134, 137
Chinese massage, 151
Chinese medicine, 3, 4–5, 10, 23–25, 58

Chinese medicine musical balls, 207, 209
Chiropractors, 8, 9
Chromotherapy. *See* Color therapy
Chronic illness, 242–43, 247
Chronic inflammation, 212–13
Chronic pain, 213–14
Circular friction, 102, 103
Circulatory system
effects of massage on, 29–30, 36
Client Financial Record, 259
Client folder forms, 255–59
Client Information Form, 260
Clients
after-massage treatment, 79–80
communication with, 72–73
determining needs of, 72–73
draping, 77–79
interaction with, 73–76
positioning, 77–79, 240–41, 261
Cocci, 45, 46
Code of ethics, 17–20, 252–53
Cold friction, 217
Cold hydrotherapy (cryotherapy), 60, 217, 218. *See also* RICE therapy
effects of, 219, 221
for inflammation, 213
techniques, 221, 222
for tendinitis, 239
uses of, 221
Color therapy, 57, 163–65
Commission on Massage Therapy Approval/Accreditation (COMTAA), 8
Communicable diseases, 47, 49
Communication
therapist-client, 72–73
Compresses, 217
Compression, 121
defined, 84–86
in neuromuscular therapy, 139
Compressive force, 103
Computerized tomography (CT), 176
Confidentiality, 19
Connective tissue
effects of massage on, 32
Connective tissue techniques, 11, 117, 127–129
Consultation, 74–75
Contagion, 47, 49
Contract, relax, and contract the opposite technique, 132
Contract and relax technique, 132

Contraindications
    for hydrotherapy, 219, 232
    for massage, 27, 28, 37–38
Contusions, 180–81
Counseling, 32
Cranial nerve, 229
Cranial–sacral techniques, 60, 117, 126–27
Crepius, 179
Cross-directional stretching, 113
Cross-fiber friction, 102
Cryotherapy. *See* Cold hydrotherapy (cryotherapy)
C stroke, 98, 100
Cupping, 107, 109, 110
Cushion, Michio Kusho, 154
Cutaneous pain, 26, 214
Cycle of dependence, 23
Cyriax, James, 8, 99, 127

Darius, King, 4
Deep breathing, 187, 190
Deep pain, 27, 214
Deep touch, 82, 94–95
Deep transverse frictioning, 127–28, 232
    for tendinitis, 239
Degenerative conditions, 36
Dependence
    cycle of, 23
Diabetes, 36
Diaphragmatic breathing, 187, 190, 191
Dicke, Elizabeth, 7, 128
Diffusers, 165
Diocles, 3
Diplomas, 16–17
Disabled persons
    massage for, 244
Disclosure, 19
Diseases. *See also specific diseases*
    microorganisms and, 44–47
Disinfectants, 44, 47–49
Do-in, 154
Draping the client, 77–79
Drop foot, 230

Eastern therapies. *See* Chinese medicine; Oriental
        therapies
Ebner, Maria, 7

Eddy, Mary Baker, 53
Edema, 30, 36, 129
Edison, Thomas, 173
Educational standards, 16
Effleurage, 2, 6, 10
Eisenberg, David, 58
Elbows
    inflammation of, 247
Elderly persons, 242–43, 247
Electric moist heat pads, 219
Electromyography (EMG), 176
Emotions, 55
Endangerment sites, 38–40
Endorphins, 26, 32, 34, 214
Energetic approaches, 11, 57–59
Energy (chi, qi), 57, 149
Energy brushing, 123
Energy channels, 149–152
Energy systems, 23–25
    effects of massage on, 33
Energy therapy, 160–69
Enkephalins, 214
Epsom salts, 223
Essential oils, 116, 165, 166–67
Ethics, 17–20, 252–53
Excretory system
    effects of massage on, 33, 36
Exhaustion, 186
Expiration (breathing), 190, 191
Extended triangle posture (yoga), 189
Exteroceptors, 110
Exudate, 28

Facial expression, 61
Facilitated positional release technique, 134, 136
Fascial kinetics, 128, 129
Fascial stretch, 103
Fascial techniques, 127–129
Fears
    of massage therapists, 17–19
Feather stroking, 96
Feet
    loss of muscle enervation in, 230
    plantar fascitis, 238
Felonies, 16
Felten, David, 55
Fever
    cold water therapy for, 221

Fibromyalgia, 60, 229
Fibrositis syndrome, 229
Field, Tiffany, 38, 60
Fight or flight response, 186
Finger pressure massage, 10
Finkelstein test, 237
Fitzgerald, William, 7
Flexibility, 190
Fluoromethane vasocoolant sprays, 221
Foam balls, 208
Fomentation pads, 219
Fomites, 47
Foot reflexology diagram, 143
Freud, Sigmund, 7
Friction stroke, 2, 10, 82
    application of, 99, 102, 103
    circular, 102, 103
    cold, 217
    cross-fiber, 102
    deep transverse, 127–28, 232, 239
    defined, 86, 88–89
    hot, 217
Frozen shoulder, 215
Fulling, 98, 99
Fumigants, 48
Functional pain, 26, 214
Fungi, 44–45

Gait, 190
Galenus (Galen), 3
Gliding stroke, 10, 120
    application of, 96–97
    defined, 83–84
    in neuromuscular therapy, 139
Golfer's elbow test, 239
Golgi tendon organs, 111–112
Golgi tendon receptors, 111
Graham, Douglas, 6
Graham, Martha, 211
Greater trochanter, 232
Greek, classical, 3
Ground substance, 128, 138
Gyroflex balls, 207, 209

Hacking, 105, 109
Hadrian, 4

Halpern, Stephen, 207
Hamstrings
    self-stretching exercises, 194, 196, 197
Hand reflexology diagram, 144
Hands
    care of, 200, 204–206, 207
Hard seeing, 59
Headache, 181–82
Head positions, 61
Healing and the Mind (Anderson), 56
Healing and the Mind (Moyers), 23–25
Healing Massage Techniques (Tappan), 8
Healing mechanisms, 22–25
    Oriental approach, 23–25
    wellness approach, 22–23
Health history, 75–76
Health History Form, 256
Health salons, 9
Heat therapy. See also Hot hydrotherapy
    effects of, 223
    moist, 215, 219
    uses of, 221, 223
Heavy percussion, 107
Herbs
    burning over tsubos, 157
Hippocrates, 3
Hips
    self-stretching exercises, 192–95
Hoffa, Albert, 6
Holistic approach, 23–25
Homeostasis, 23, 32
Homer, 1
HOPS assessment tool, 175–76, 179
Hoshino, 57
Hot friction, 217
Hot hydrotherapy, 217. See also Heat therapy
    for inflammation, 213
Hot tubs, 217
Hydrocollators, 219
Hydrotherapy, 2, 7, 10, 117, 216–25. See also
        Cold hydrotherapy (cryotherapy); Hot hy-
        drotherapy
    for bursitis, 228
    for chronically diseases, 243
    contraindications, 219, 232
    defined, 216
    for sprains, 227
    for strains, 226
    types of, 217
    for whiplash, 234

Ice packs, 217, 218
Immobility, 36
Immune system, 186
India, 3
Indications, 35–36
Infant massage, 38, 240–41
    routine for, 262–63
Inflammation, 28, 179
    acute, 212–13
    bursitis, 227–229
    chronic, 212–13
    of the elbow, 247
    subacute, 212–13
    systemic, 213
    therapeutic massage for, 212–13
Inflammatory arthritis, 36
Informed consent, 19
Ingham, Eunice D., 7
Injuries
    cold water therapy for, 221
Inspiration (breathing), 190, 191
Integrated approaches, 11, 170
Integrated neuromuscular inhibition (INIT), 134
Interoceptors, 110
Intractable pain, 214
Ironing, 120
Ischemia, 27
Ischial tuberosity, 232
Isokinetic contractions, 131
Isokinetic evaluation, 176
Isometric contractions, 131
Isotonic contractions, 131

Jacuzzi, 217
Japan, 10
Joint movement, 87
Joint play technique, 120
Jones, Lawrence, 132
Journaling, 207

Kellogg, John H., 6
Kenny, Sister, 7
Ki. *See* Chi
Kleer, Enril Andrea Gabriel, 6
Kneading strokes, 10, 82
    application of, 97–101

defined, 84–85
variations of, 98, 100–101, 104

Latex gloves, 49
Latissimus dorsi muscle, 119
Lengthening, 113–115
Licensing, 8–9, 15–17
    for acupuncture, 154
Lief, Stanley, 139
Light touch, 82, 93
Linens, 49
Ling, Per Henrik, 5, 82
Ling system, 5
Liver disease, 30
Local cold application, 217, 218
Local conditions
    with contraindications for massage, 37
Local heat application, 217
Local inflammation, 28
Longitudinal stretching, 113–114
Low back
    self-stretching exercises, 192–94
Lowen, Alexander, 7
Lucas-Champronniere, Marie, 6
Lymphatic drainage, 11
Lymphatic massage, 60
Lymphatic system
    effects of massage on, 30–31, 36
Lymph nodes, 30–31
Lymphocytes, 30

Magnetic resonance imaging (MRI), 176
Mainstream approach, 56–57, 59
Make a heart technique, 263
Manual lymphatic drainage, 8, 30–31, 128–30
Manual lymph drainage strokes, 120
Manual of Hydrotherapy and Massage, 217
Mary, Queen of Scots, 4
Massage. *See also* Swedish massage; Therapeutic
        massage; *specific massage strokes*
    atmosphere for, 70–72
    for Bell's palsy, 230
    benefits of, 63–66
    for bursitis, 227–229
    for carpal tunnel syndrome, 238
    contemporary approaches, 126–71

Massage (*cont.*)
  contraindications, 27, 28, 37–38
  current modalities, 10–12
  current research, 35
  defined, 2, 14
  emotional effects of, 34–35
  for fibromyalgia (fibrositis syndrome), 229
  future of, 9–10
  history of, 3–7
  indications for, 35–36
  origins of word, 2
  physiologic effects of, 28–33
  for piriform syndrome, 230–33
  primary benefits, 36
  psychological effects of, 33–34
  for sciatic nerve, 230–33
  secondary benefits, 36
  spiritual effects of, 34–35
  for sprains, 226–227
  for strains, 225–226
  strokes, 2, 6, 81–124, 82–92, 93–109
  for whiplash, 233–34
Massage and Therapeutic Exercise (McMillan), 7
Massage Therapy Journal, 70
Mastectomy, 37, 245–46
McMillan, Mary, 7
Meditation tapes, 206–207
Meridians, 23–24, 149
Metazoans, 45
Mezger, J. G., 6
Microorganisms, 44–47
Middle Ages, 4
Mills, Charles, 6
Mind-body relationship, 54–59
Minsky Marvin, 81
Moist heat, 215, 219
Moxa, 157
Moxibustion, 157
Moyers, Bill, 23–25, 56–57
MRI, 176
Mugwort, 158
Multiple sclerosis, 246–47
Muscle contractions, 131
Muscle energy techniques (METs), 113, 131–37
Muscle pain, 27
Muscle spindle cells, 110–111
Muscle testing, 120, 176–78
Muscular system
  effects of massage on, 33
Myelograms, 176

Myofascial pain, 60
Myofascial release, 120
  for tendinitis, 239
Myofascial techniques, 137–39, 140, 144, 146
Myotherapy, 146

National Certification Board for Therapeutic Massage and Bodywork (NCBTMB), 8–9, 16–17
  Code of Ethics, 252–53
National Certification Proficiency Examination, 16
Natural Healing with Water, Herbs, and Sunlight, 217
Neck, 66
Necrosis, 28
Nerve stroking, 96
Nervous system
  effects of massage on, 31–32
Neuromuscular techniques, 11, 120–121, 139–48
Nociceptors, 25
Norepinephrine, 26, 214
Nursing homes
  massage in, 242–43, 247

Objective assessment, 174–75
Ohashi, 155
Ohashi Institute, 155
One-handed kneading, 98
Orbital vibrator, 105
Oriental therapies, 11, 23–25, 121, 149–158
Ornish, Dean, 55
Orthobionomy, 139, 141
Oscillating vibrator, 105
Osler, William, 69

Pain, 25–28
  acute, 213
  chronic, 213–214
  components of, 25
  cutaneous, 214
  defined, 213
  functional (psychogenic), 214
  intractable (deep), 214
  massage for, 213–16, 215, 244
  phantom, 214, 216
  referred, 214, 215, 216

responses to, 214
sources of, 26, 214
transmission of, 112
types of, 27
visceral, 214
Pain killers, 28
Pain–spasm–pain cycle, 26–27
Pain threshold, 25, 93, 96
Palpation, 76, 175
    for bursitis, 228
    for strains, 226
    for tendinitis, 239
    for whiplash, 234
Parasympathetic nervous system, 32
Parasympathetic response, 187
Paré, Ambroise, 4
Paresthesia, 221
Parker, Johnny, 241
Passive positioning methods, 141
Passive rhythmic movements (Trager®), 121
Pathogens, 44–477
Pauls, Arthur Lincoln, 139
Peijian, Shen, 151
Pelvis movement, 61
Percussion strokes, 10, 86, 90–91, 105–111
Personal hygiene, 50–51
Personal Information and Financial Agreement,
    257
Pert, Candace, 56–57
Pettrisage, 2, 6, 10
Phalen's test, 236
Phantom pain, 214
Physical fitness movement, 8
Physiology, 54
Piezoelectric current, 137–38
Piriformis
    self-stretching exercises, 194, 197
Piriform syndrome, 230–33
Piriform test, 230
Pitting edema, 30
Plantar fasciitis, 238
Platysma, 215
Pliny, 4
Polarity therapy, 11, 160, 162, 163
Polarity Therapy Association, 160
Positional release (PR), 11, 113
Positional release/strain–counterstrain technique,
    134, 135
Positioning, 77–79
    for pregnant clients, 77, 240–41, 261

Postevent massage, 242
Postural integration, 11, 160
Posture
    assessment/body reading, 59–66
    balanced and imbalanced, 179
    correction exercises, 190–92
Practitioners. *See also* Therapist-client interaction
    burnout in, 187–88
Pre-event massage, 242
Pregnancy
    massage in, 240–41
    massage routine, 261–62
    positioning, 77, 240–4, 261–62
Pressure points, 155
Professional demeanor, 19–20
Proprioception, 110–113
Proprioceptive neuromuscular facilitation (PNF),
    113–114, 131, 232
Prorioceptors, 110
Protozoa, 45
Prudden, Bonnie, 8, 144
Pseudomonas, 45
Psoas
    self-stretching exercises, 196, 198
Psychogenic pain, 26
Psychological pain, 214
Psychoneuroimmunology, 54
Pulsed muscle energy procedures, 134
Putty balls, 207

Qi. *See* Chi

Range-of-motion (ROM)
    movements, 14
    tests, 175–76, 179
Receptors, 110
Reciprocal inhibition technique, 132, 133
Reference library, 38
Referrals, 41–42
    for pain, 215
    for testing procedures, 176
Referred pain, 27, 146, 214, 215
Reflexology, 7, 27, 121, 122, 143–44, 145
Rehabilitation massage, 242
Reich, Wilhelm, 7
Reiki, 163

Relaxation tapes, 206–207
Relaxation techniques, 117
Repetitive exercise, 64–65
Resistance response, 186
Resistive range-of-motion (ROM) tests, 176
Respiratory system
    effects of massage on, 32
Rest homes
    massage in, 242–43, 257
Restorative massage, 242
Rhazes (Razi), 4
Rib cage compression, 61
RICE (rest, ice, compression, and elevation),
        121–22, 213, 223
Rickettsiae, 45, 47
Right of refusal, 19
Right-sidedness, 61
Rocking techniques, 105, 107
Rolf, Ida, 160
Rolfing®, 11, 160
Rolf Institute, 160
Roman empire, 3–4
Roth, Mathias, 5
Routines, 178
Rubber balls, 208
Russia, 10
Russian baths, 220

Safe environment, 70–72
Safe touch, 19
Safety practices, 49, 50
    in animal massage, 169
Salmonella, 45
Salt baths, 223
Salt glow, 217
Sanitation practices, 47–49
Sauna, 217
Scandals, 6
Sciatic nerve, 230–33
Scope of practice, 14
Sea products, 225
Seated massage, 72, 73, 122, 159, 182–83
Sedative massage techniques, 32
Self-care activities, 185–209
    for burnout, 188
    deep breathing exercises, 190
    hands and arms, 200, 204–206
    postural correction exercises, 190–92

relaxation, meditation, and visualization tapes,
        206–207
    stretching, 190–200, 201–203
    Tai chi, 189–90
    touch for health, 206–207
    for whiplash, 234
    yoga, 189
Selye, Hans, 34, 186
Seminar Network International School of Massage,
        38
Seneca, 3–4
Sexual impropriety, 19
Shaking techniques, 105, 106
Shamans, 3
Shea, Michael, 126
Shepard, Paul, 185
Shiatsu, 10, 154–57
Shoulders, 66
    frozen, 215
    position, 61
    self-stretching exercises, 196, 200–202, 204
Showers, 217
Skin rolling, 98, 121
    in neuromuscular therapy, 139
Slapping, 107, 109
SOAP notes, 76–77, 174–75
SOAP Reporting Form, 258
Soft seeing, 59
Soft tissue, 14
Somatic Release, 57
Somatic structures, 26
Sound therapy, 163, 165
Soviet Sports Review Journal, 241
Spas, 4, 9–10, 217
Spasticity
    of spinal chord injuries, 64
Special populations, 38
    massage for, 38
    therapeutic massage for, 240–44
Speech
    neck and, 66
Speed's test, 240
Spinal chord injuries, 64
Spindle cells, 110–111
Spirilla, 45, 46
Spirit, 55
Sports injuries
    RICE for, 223
Sports massage, 84–85, 241–42, 246
Sprains, 226–227

Spray-and-stretch, 117, 118
Spray and stretch technique, 134, 137
Sprays, 217
St. John, Paul, 139
Stabbing pain, 27
Staphylococci, 44, 45
Steam, 217
Steam cabinet baths, 220
Steam cabinets, 220
Stone, Randolph, 160
Stories the Feet Tell (Ingham), 7
Strain–counterstrain (SCS) techniques, 11, 113,
    122–23, 134, 135
Strains, 225–226
Streptococci, 44, 45
Stress, 186–87, 186–187
    burnout and, 187–88
    massage for, 246
    pain and, 34
    stages of, 186
Stress–pain–stress cycle, 34
StressTouch therapy, 65
Stretching, 113–115, 121, 190–200, 201–203
    ballistic, 192
    general principles, 192
    in neuromuscular therapy, 139
    self-stretching exercises, 192–200
Stroking techniques, 123. *See also under Massage;*
    specific strokes
Stroking the aura, 160
Structural alignment technique, 11, 65, 160
Structural positioning, 123
Students
    burnout in, 187–88
Subacute inflammation, 212–13
Subjective Assessment, 174
Subliminal tapes, 207
Sun moon technique, 263
Suppuration, 28
Sutherland, William, 126
Swedish massage, 5, 10, 123–24, 129
    defined, 2
    physiological effects of, 29–30
    in pregnancy, 240–41
    for tendinitis, 239
Swedish shampooing, 217
Sympathetic nervous system, 32
Systemic conditions
    with contraindications for massage, 37
Systemic inflammation, 28, 213

Tai chi, 189–90
Tapotement, 2, 6, 10
Tappan, Francis, 8
Tapping, 107
Taylor, Charles Fayette, 5
Taylor, George Henry, 6
T-bars, 142, 146
Technik der Massage (Hoffa), 6
Temporomandibular joint (TMJ), 66, 182–83
Tendinitis, 212, 238–40
Tennis elbow test, 239
Tense and relax technique, 132
Tension, 186–87, 186–187
    burnout and, 187–88
10-zone theory, 143
Terminally ill patients, 244
Textbook of Orthopedic Medicine (Cyriax), 8
Thai massage, 57, 157–58
Thalassotherapy, 225
Therapeutic massage, 211–47
    defined, 14
    for inflammation, 212–13
    for pain, 213–16
    for special populations, 240–44
Therapeutic touch, 57, 163. *See also* Touch
    benefits of, 66
Therapist-client interaction. *See also* Practitioners
    communication, 72–73
    guidelines for, 70–72, 73–76
Therapy room setup, 70–72
Thumper, 105
Tinel's test, 236–37
Tissue injury, 212
Touch, 2, 10. *See also* Therapeutic touch
    application of, 93–96
    benefits of, 60
    defined, 82
    physiological effects of, 93
Touch for health, 207, 209
Touch Research Institute, 60
Toxin removal
    heat therapy for, 221, 223
Trager, Milton, 146
Trager® technique, 121, 146–49
Trauma victims, 244
Travell, Janet, 144
Treatment plans, 76–77
Trigger points, 116, 141, 144, 146, 147, 215
Trigger point therapy, 221
Tsubos, 10, 151, 154

Uttihita trikon asana, 189

Vectors, 47
Vibrational therapies, 2, 10, 36, 160–69
    application of, 102–105
    for Bell's palsy, 245
    defined, 86 92
Vibrators, 105
Viruses, 45, 47
Visceral pain, 26, 214
Visualization tapes, 206–207
Vodder, Emil, 8, 129
Vodder lymph drainage, 129
V stroke, 98, 100

Warm-down period, 192
Warm-up period, 192
Water wheel technique, 263
Weight management, 36
Wellness, 22–23, 185–209
    burnout and, 188
Western medicine, 23
Wheelchair massage, 247

Whiplash
    massage for, 233–34
Whirlpool baths, 217
Whole person
    treating, 54–56
Wrist
    carpal tunnel syndrome, 235–38
Writing
    in journals, 207

X-rays, 176

Yang, 23–25, 149
Yang channels, 150–53
Yanni, 207
Yessi, Michael, 241
Yin, 23–25, 149
Yin channels, 150–53
Yoga, 189

Zone therapy, 7, 143–44, 145